African American Women's Health and Social Issues

African American Women's Health and Social Issues

SECOND EDITION

Edited by Catherine Fisher Collins

Foreword by Vivian W. Pinn

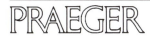

PRAEGER

Westport, Connecticut
London

This book is dedicated to the late Herman Fisher Jr. I love you and I miss you.

Your Sister

This book is also dedicated to my friend the late Mrs. Barbara Bowman Penn of Timmonsville, South Carolina. I miss your beautiful smile and your compassionate heart.

Your Friend

Library of Congress Cataloging-in-Publication Data

African American women's health and social issues / edited by Catherine Fisher Collins.—2nd ed.
    p. cm.
  Includes bibliographical references and index.
  ISBN 0–275–98082–0 (alk. paper)
  1. African American women—Health and hygiene. 2. African American women—
Diseases. 3. African American women—Social conditions. I. Collins, Catherine Fisher.
  RA448.5.N4A445 2006
  613'.0424408996073—dc22   2006008227

British Library Cataloguing in Publication Data is available.

This book is included in the African American Experience database from Greenwood Electronic
Media. For more information, visit www.africanamericanexperience.com.

Library of Congress Catalog Card Number: 2006008227
ISBN: 0–275–98082–0

First published in 2006

Praeger Publishers, 88 Post Road West, Westport, CT 06881
An imprint of Greenwood Publishing Group, Inc.
www.praeger.com

Printed in the United States of America

The paper used in this book complies with the
Permanent Paper Standard issued by the National
Information Standards Organization (Z39.48–1984).

10 9 8 7 6 5 4 3 2 1

Contents

Foreword

VIVIAN W. PINN, M.D.

Ten years ago when I wrote the foreword to the first edition of this book, the concept of women's health was changing at a rapid pace. The focus was just shifting from solely reproductive issues and biological factors, to an expanded perception that women's health encompasses biological, familial, cultural, economic, emotional, psychological, and behavioral elements of each woman and her sociopolitical environment, beyond just the reproductive organs and across her entire lifespan. This rapid pace has continued and been magnified as our research and advocacy efforts have garnered new information and deeper and broader insights into women's health as a totality.

Furthermore, we now have new information about the health of African American women and the factors that influence their health. Much of that documentation and data have resulted because of policies that have required epidemiologic and biomedical researchers to pay specific attention to the health issues of ethnic and racial population groups and of women as well as men. At the National Institutes of Health, the Office of Research on Women's Health has been the focal point for ensuring that policies, which require the inclusion of women and minorities in clinical research, are fully implemented and that research studies are designed so that information from such studies can benefit the diversity of the public health community, including African American women. A second important stimulus for new and better information has been a movement among women, especially women of color, in the biomedical and social sciences, health professions, policy fields, and media to give voice to the specific health issues of African American women. *African American Women's Health and Social Issues, Second Edition* is a significant illustration of this stimulus.

With knowledge and insights come opportunities and responsibilities, and unless we embrace those opportunities and responsibilities as a society and as individuals, the knowledge remains mere data, the insights good intentions. I commend the authors of the chapters in this book for presenting not only the data relevant to their subjects and then also to African American women, but for addressing the issues of how we can personally take steps to improve our own health—whether by adopting pro-health behaviors or by becoming more informed and clever about accessing the health care system to meet our needs.

The numerical data—statistics on death, disease rates, utilization of the health care system—help us to understand where we as policymakers, health care professionals, and individuals of concerned awareness must focus our efforts and our knowledge. These numbers and percentages are guideposts, even red flags, that lead policymakers to support biomedical research that reveal the factors that cause the health problems and present barriers to health care, and where public health policymakers determine where new policies and procedures are needed to lessen and eliminate health disparities. Those factors are sometimes genetic, sometimes biologically infectious conditions. Often they are cultural, attitudinal, behavioral, sociopolitical, or socioeconomic conditions that exacerbate disease, predispose individuals to disease, or interfere with health care delivery. Those factors also might affect the patient and they might affect the health care professional, but knowing what the factors are is the first step in changing them.

The data presented in these chapters can empower us by showing us what our risks, as African American women, are and what to expect. Forewarned is forearmed if we have the commitment to act in our own best interests. Each individual must consider her own health in terms of her own circumstances. What are the stumbling blocks for our own health, and what are the barriers to having better health for us? Are the barriers real or perceived? What personal actions can we take to better utilize the health care system? What personal behaviors do we need to adopt to stay healthy—a more healthful diet, weight control, more physical activity, stress reduction, safe sex, medical or dental checkups? I urge you to use the data to stimulate your commitment to do more for yourself, your children, and your grandchildren. Advice on how to do so is in each chapter of this book.

We, as African American women, are not alone in these efforts. Attention to the role of social and biological factors, and gender factors, in health and disease has taken hold not only across the United States, but in many nations around the world. Ten years from now, surely we will look back and see that the concepts of preserving wellness and preventing diseases will have changed worldwide to embrace the roles of many elements of society, at the same time influencing public health policymakers, researchers, health care professionals, individual women and their families, and communities to be better enabled to have a longer and healthier lives. As African American women, we can derive energy from knowing that others are working to learn our needs, helping us to meet our needs, and keeping a positive perspective. At the same time, we need to use our energy to take care of ourselves. Then, in ten years, we can rejoice in witnessing a positive trend in improved health for African American women.

Preface

The African American women who are the contributors of the thirteen chapters you are about to read are caring and knowledgeable about the negative social and health issues that plague their communities. For too "many years the literatures on these issues have been dominated by white male writers, followed by white females and black males, who all believe that they know what we want, when we know that the best authority about us—is us" (Collins, 1996, p. xvii).

First, you will experience a commentary on the current health status and social conditions of African American women, as seen through the eyes and experiences of the editor, followed by thirteen dynamic and informative chapters.

Chapter 1 presents heart disease—one of the most insidious diseases affecting the health of African American women, and their number one killer. To demonstrate the seriousness of this disease, research from various authorities is cited, including a recent study by the American Heart Association. Also well documented in this chapter is the devastating effect caused when heart disease combines with other factors such as a sedentary lifestyle, or diseases like diabetes or hypertension. How to survive the effects of heart disease is also discussed.

Chapter 2 addresses the issue of breast cancer, examining some of the important factors believed to be linked to the disproportionately high disease rate among African American females. Also of great concern is the impact of racism on their poor survival rate. In the early 1980s, there was a flurry of social concerns regarding sickle cell disease. In Chapter 3, the physical and psychosocial aspects of sickle cell disease (SCD) across the life span are discussed, highlighting reproductive concerns and issues during pregnancy. Also discussed is an historical recounting of the discovery of SCD, as well as the influences of racism, stigma, and discrimination toward African American women. Some treatment options are presented, and the need is expressed for increased awareness that will help

African American women make responsible decisions. Unlike the 1980s, when there was a burst of information regarding the origin of sickle cell and social concerns for African Americans, these issues appeared to fade. Therefore, in this chapter the author presents a reexamination of this chronic illness and its impact on the African American female. Chapter 4 presents further insights. Also addressed in both Chapters 3 and 4 is a discussion on the origin of SDC.

One in four African American women over 55 years of age has diabetes, the subject of Chapter 5. It is estimated that there are over 13 million Americans with some form of diabetes, and African American women who are overweight are predisposed to this ravaging illness. This chapter also addresses lifestyle and cultural influences, and how the church has developed health programs that are documenting measurable successes in attacking diabetes.

HIV/AIDS, and the basic factors that contribute to the victimization of African American women across socioeconomic lines by this most devastating disease, are the subject of Chapter 6. Health indicators will be shared to help the reader better understand the critical urgency for African American women to take control of their sexuality. Chapter 7 addresses the social consequences of HIV/AIDS. This chapter explores the conceptualization that transmission of the disease goes beyond the use of condoms and behavior, to a deeper level of internal motivators of behaviors. Another look at the impact of HIV/AIDS on the African American female population is presented in Chapter 8. The discussion reveals that this disease—which has escalated into a pandemic—continues to affect women worldwide and, in the United States, African American women in particular.

In Chapter 9, mental health issues among African American women are brought to light through a review of the literature for relevant studies on this subject. The problem of depression among African American women is well documented here.

Chapter 10 is an exploration of the complex plight of homeless African American women. This chapter documents the growth of America's homeless population, while focusing on the group with largest growth—single mothers with children.

The central theme of Chapter 11 is showing how important Informed Consent is to the survival of African American women. African American women must be responsible for knowing what power they are giving to others when asked to give consent. This chapter explains the need to be informed.

Chapter 12 presents a subject on which most literature has been silent: how African American girls are socialized in America's Catholic schools. Catholic school education is shown to have had a somewhat negative impact on Black womanhood, affecting the ability to cope.

The final chapter, Chapter 13, explores the coping ability of African American women, presenting how they have been able to survive the social ills of America and describing their coping styles.

Acknowledgments

There are so many to thank, but I must first begin with the Almighty—Thanks Be to God.

Once again this book would not have been possible were it not for the "Sisters," who made it possible. To each of the Sisters/Contributors—Virginia A. Batchelor, Lynne Valencia Perry-Bottinger, Patricia K. Bradley, Renee Bowman Daniels, Cassandra Dobson, Imani Lillie B. Fryar, Cheryl Hunter-Grant, Juanita K. Hunter, Jamesetta A. Newland, Freida Outlaw, Lorraine E. Peeler, Rhea J. Simmons—your commitment to seeing this book to its fruition is far beyond a thank-you. To Dr.Vivian Pinn, I once again thank you for your continuous support and for contributing the foreword. My wonderful parents, the late Herman and Catherine Fisher—I love and miss you. My daughter, Laura Harris, and son, Dr. Clyde A Collins II, you are the loves of my life; how do I thank you for being my children? My colleagues at the State University of New York, Empire State College, and other colleagues at the State University of New York Women's Studies Department, your support is appreciated—thank you. I thank Sami M. Cirpili for his technical graphic assistance. To my friends in Jack and Jill of America, Inc., and to members of the Buffalo Public School Board, For Women Only, and The Buffalo Links, Inc.—thank you. And last, to everyone that I missed, know that you are all very special in my life and this book.

Introduction: Commentary on the Health and Social Status of African American Women

CATHERINE FISHER COLLINS

Since my 1996 commentary on the health and social status of African American women, the disparity that exists among these women has had minimal improvement. A review of the literature and the data contained in this second edition is proof that there is much that needs to be done in order to elevate these women to the level of health and social status experienced by their white counterparts. This commentary is designed to explore some of the health and social conditions that negatively impact African American women.

We know that some illnesses are fueled by social problems such as racism, while others are due to environment, poverty, low levels of education, and poor lifestyle choices such as smoking, drug use, and unprotected sex. In seeking to understand how sick a population really is, life expectancy and mortality data are two indications of a population's state of health.

Life expectancy "describes the likelihood of surviving to a given age at a given time in history" (Harper & Lambert, 1994, p. 16). Life expectancy is not only about how long African American women are expected to live, but it is also a good indication of how they are meeting the enormous challenges of society, as compared to other women. Unfortunately, the optimal health of a population is standardized by whom the county designates as the healthiest. Therefore, for this commentary, white American women will be our comparative population. Although some Asian women are healthier on some health indicators (Leigh & Jimenez, 2003, pp. ix, 55), white women are usually used as the comparative grouping studies of African American women. As previously mentioned, data on life expectancy is important and, in my estimation, an important indicator of how African American women are doing. An examination of this data reveals that African American women's health continues to lag behind that of white women (Table I.1). In 1900, white women lived an average of 48.7 years while

Table I.1
Life expectancy 1960–2001 of African American and White Women

Race	1960*	1970*	1980*	1990**	1992**	2001***
White American	74.1	75.6	78.7	79.4	79.7	79.9
African American	66.3	68.3	72.5	73.6	73.9	74.7

Source: Wegman, M. December 1990* and 1992**, Table 4, p. 841*, Table 4, p. 747**, U.S. Department of Health and Human Services, Office on Women's Health Issues, 2004, p. 7.***

African American women lived an average of 33.5. Today, the life-expectancy gap continues, showing a very poor outlook for African American women.

Mortality data also tells us how well African American women are surviving and what's killing them off. The numbers speak for themselves: The overall mortality rate of white women in 1998 was 372.5 per 100,000, while the rate for African American women was 589.4 per 100,000 (Misra, 2000, p. 65). Needless to say, African American women are not doing well in comparison to their white counterparts.

The media and other sources often present information in such a way that leads others to conclude that African American woman and poor women receive considerable health resources, driving up Medicaid health care costs. However, what often isn't stated is that there are currently 46 million uninsured Americans (Wallechinsky, 2005, p. 4) and that even though Medicaid is this nation's health insurance program for the poor and low income, it is means-tested. In other words, if an applicant fails to meet the eligibility requirements—and being poor does not automatically qualify one for Medicaid coverage—then the applicant typically joins the ranks of the uninsured.

The Institute of Medicine "concluded that providing health insurance to uninsured adults would result in improved health, including greater life expectancy. In particular, increasing the rate of health insurance coverage would especially improve the health of those in the poorest health and most disadvantaged in terms of access to care and thus would likely reduce health disparities among racial and ethnic groups" (U.S. Department of Health and Human Services [DHHS], 2003, p. 112). Further, the "National Academy of Science estimates that 18,000 adults die each year because they are uninsured and cannot get proper care" (*New York Times*, 5/29/05, p. 19).

According to Weisman (2002), at the end of 2001 there were "34.6 million Americans who lived in poverty. . . . The poverty rate rose for the second straight year to 12.1 percent in 2002 from 11.7 percent the year before [and the poor] were concentrated among African Americans, suburban residents and Midwesterners" (p. 1).

When people are poor they fail to seek health care for two reasons: no health insurance and inability to pay for health care (Leigh & Jimenez, 2003, p. ix). African American women have more undetected diseases and chronic and acute illnesses than other women (Leigh & Jimenez, 2003, pp. 17–18). Some of these illnesses may be due to not having health insurance or means to pay for it, while others may be due to lifestyle behaviors (e.g., alcoholism, drug use) or genetics (glaucoma, sickle cell) that may affect life expectancy.

Furthermore, when poverty is facilitated by racism, disease states flourish. For example, a look at the historical context of service delivery pre-1900 finds meager health care was offered to sick female slaves or free Black women. Their poor health condition led F. L. Hoffman to state, in his book, *Race Traits and Tendencies of the American Negro*, that Blacks showed the least ability to compete in the struggle for existence (p. 148), and that this was justification to do nothing about the health needs of African Americans. As a result, African American women learned early on to endure many illnesses without proper health care, dying at an alarming rate from childbirth and other preventable health conditions. With limited access to hospital delivery rooms in the 1930s, some mothers survived. However, tuberculosis (TB) and syphilis held back any substantial gains, thus contributing to morbidity.

Following the end of World War I, limited gains in health conditions were experienced by African American women (Beardsley, 1990). The Great Depression served as the force that essentially eliminated some of the public health clinics and programs. It was not until the passage of the 1935 Social Security Act that some clinics in poor neighborhoods were reestablished. Later, African American women could seek care in the free public health clinics and hospitals created by the Hill Burton Act of 1946. Under Hill Burton, hospitals were more willing to allow African American women to deliver in hospitals once reserved for white women even if the bed was unoccupied. As more African American women sought hospital care, it became very apparent that racism was not confined to their neighborhoods. A well-devised and -defined, segregated health care delivery system developed, one for Blacks and one for whites. This segregated health care system was challenged by the National Association for the Advancement of Colored People (NAACP), and the overt discrimination in health care became less distinguishable because of potential loss of federal funding and the ability to sue under the Civil Rights Act of 1964.

However, even with better access to health care, African American women remain the sickest of American citizens. Gaining access is no guarantee that what is needed is what will be provided. Furthermore, having insurance is no guarantee that the service African American women receive is equal to that provided for their white counterparts. This inequality was described in a *Health-Quest* article, which reported that "studies show that doctors routinely give Black patients outmoded therapies, second-best medications and inferior services compared with Whites, even when the patients have comparable incomes" ("State of Black Health Care," 2001, p. 25). To demonstrate the inequality, the article states: "In one recent study of over 600 physician-patient encounters at 10 New York state hospitals, cardiologists admitted that they viewed Black patients as less intelligent than Whites, and poor patients as less rational than [nonpoor] Whites, even though both groups of patients had similar psychological profiles" (p. 25). Also, when medical education fails to provide training in cultural competencies and patients are treated with disrespect, it lowers their satisfaction with the care they have received—a possible contributing factor to low rates of follow-up visits. Indeed, Meadows (2005) said: "If you think the race or ethnicity of doctor plays no role in the quality of your health, think again. Nearly one-third of the U.S. population is at risk of lost productivity, pain and suffering or even worse, premature death, simply because they don't have a doctor who looks like or can relate to them" (p. 106). Combined, African Americans, Latinos, and Native Americans make up 25 percent of the population (Johnson, 2004–5, p. 106). However, they make up only 6 percent of physicians, 9 percent of nurses, and 5 percent of dentists. If these numbers are not bleak enough, in the health professional schools, people of color make up only 4.2 percent of medical schools, 8.5 percent of dental schools, and 10 percent of the baccalaureate nursing faculties. These disparities are discussed later, and will show that the absence of people of color in the health care profession, coupled with lack of health insurance and access to health care, only add to the problems that plague African American women.

African Americans are often reminded of the Tuskegee syphilis experiment unauthorized by the U.S. public health service, which sought to learn more about how syphilis actually attacked the body and how treatment of 400 men, all poor, all Black was withheld, and reported wrong leg amputation of an African American (Collins, 1996). With these and other historical accounts of the mistreatment of African Americans, coupled with racist providers, some would justify a skipped follow-up appointment or disregard a sore that will not heal.

As if the lack of health insurance, lack of access, racism, and poverty were not enough, lifestyle behaviors of African American women also seriously affect their health status and longevity. Illnesses are sometimes caused by inappropriate health habits and lifestyle behaviors, which makes these women more susceptible to a variety of illnesses. Many illnesses are preventable, including diabetes type 2, which is predisposed by obesity. In 2000 "more than three-quarters (78%) of African American women between the ages of 20 and 74 were classified overweight and 50.8% were classified obese (DHHS, 2004, p. 9). Also prevalent are lung and throat cancer, which are related to smoking; cardiovascular diseases, which are often predisposed by high cholesterol; and cirrhosis of the liver, which is predisposed by alcohol consumption and drug addition. These illnesses are preventable, yet each has a devastating effect on the health status of African American females.

In the case of drug-addicted behavior, the health status of African American women is further compromised by exposure to a variety of sexually transmitted diseases (STDs) that occur in the general population at an estimated "15 million . . . cases a year—higher than any developed country" (Misra, 2000, p. 46).

Chlamydia (caused by *Chlamydia trachomatis*) is a devastating STD that is ravaging African American women in the 15–24 year age group (Misra, 2000, p. 47). The treatment of women affected with Chlamydia is extremely important since, if left untreated, this disease can cause pelvic inflammatory disease (PID). Pelvic inflammatory disease may affect the fallopian tubes, causing scarring. This predisposes women to ectopic pregnancy, which can be fatal. In 1989, the death rate from ectopic pregnancy among African Americans was 5 times higher than among white women (Horton, 1995, p. 17).

Figure I.1
Black Females as a Percentage of the U.S. Female Population

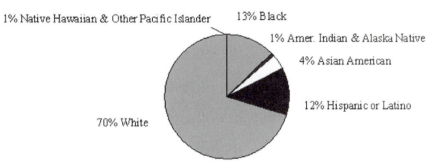

1% Native Hawaiian & Other Pacific Islander   13% Black

1% Amer. Indian & Alaska Native

4% Asian American

12% Hispanic or Latino

70% White

Source: U.S. Department of Health and Human Services (2004, p. 2).

Gonorrhea cases in 1999 totaled 360,076 in the United States, of which 179,534 were women. Of these women affected, a majority—75 percent—were African American. Thus, African American women are disproportionately represented among gonorrhea cases, as they make up only 13 percent of the U.S. female population (see Figure I.1). When you compare the number of individual reported cases in 1999, African American women cases were 764 per 100,000 and white women were 34 per 100,000 (Leigh & Jimenez, 2003, p. 109).

In 2000 a slight decline in gonorrhea was reported for both men and women (Misra, 2000, p. 49). However, according to Misra, "Regardless of declines, gonorrhea is still common within high-density urban areas among persons less than 24 years old, those who have multiple sexual partners and those who engage in unprotected sexual intercourse" (2000, p. 50). Moreover, chlamydia and gonorrhea are not the only STDs making an impact. As of 1999, whereas chlamydia affected 3–4 million people, human papillomavirus (HPV) impacted 20 million people (DHHS, 2003, p. 2); Hepatitis B, (HVB) 200,000; HIV/AIDS, up to 900,000 (Misra, 2000, p. 47–55); Genital Herpes (HSV-2), "65 million people living with it in the United States and 15 million new cases a year" (DHHS, 2004, p. 19). These escalating STD rates are having a devastating effect on the health of African American women. Indeed, Delbanco (2004) reporting on HPV, which has become one of the most common STDs in the United States, noted, "Three out of every four people will get the virus at some point in their lives [and] HPV leads to 99.7 percent of cases of cervical cancer" (p. 110). This is a disease with no known cure. These infectious diseases, when combined with poor lifestyle behavioral choices, are particularly threatening to the health of African American women.

The lifestyle choices of some African American women—and resulting behaviors—are responsible for some of their major illnesses. As previously mentioned, many of the infectious STDs are those which have a behavioral component that, for most of them, can be prevented if behavior was altered, such as use of condoms during sex. Unfortunately, condoms can't offer 100 percent

Table I.2
Ten Leading Causes of Death in African American and White Women, 1999

African American	White Women
Heart disease	Heart disease
Malignant neoplasms	Malignant neoplasms
Cerebrovascular disease	Cerebrovascular disease
Diabetes	Chronic lower respirator
Unintentional injuries	Pneumonia/Influenza
Nephritis, Nephrotic, Nephrosis Diseases	Alzheimer
Chronic lower respiratory, Unintentional Injuries	Unintentional injuries
Septicemia	Diabetes
Pneumonia/Influenza	Nephritis, Nephrotic, Nephrosis Diseases
HIV/Disease	Septicemia

Source: Leigh, W. & Jimenez, M. (2003, table 3, p. 59).

protection, and use of one won't protect the user against HPV (Delbano, p. 110). Similarly, other illnesses have a lifestyle/behavior component that place the African American female health status in jeopardy. One such illness among African American women that has a higher prevalence because of lifestyle is diabetes type 2. As shown in Table I.2, diabetes is the fourth-leading cause of death among African American females.

African American women with diabetes have an increased risk of developing heart, kidney, peripheral vascular, and eye diseases as well as complications during pregnancy. In 1997 loss of life for African American women with diabetes was 318.3 per 100,000 as compared to white females whose rate was 111.1 per 100,000. Women have been forewarned that "primary prevention of type 2 diabetes ... may be achieved through maintenance of ideal body weight over the courses of a woman's lifetime ... control of blood glucose levels and maintenance of normal body weight through diet and exercise" (Maris, p. 74). Also reported by Maris, women who are overweight and have diabetes have a two-fold increased risk of developing endometreal cancer (p. 74).

As previously mentioned, heart disease is a problem for women with diabetes and is two to four times more likely in women with diabetes (Collins, 1996, p. 5). Some doctors believe that there may be a link between heart disease and gynecological problems. African American women have more external fibroid tumors and undergo more hysterectomies, both of which can cause damage to the estrogen producing ovaries and leave the heart somewhat vulnerable.

As shown in Table I.3, in 1999 heart disease was the leading cause of death in both African American and white females as compared to cancer rates.

Risk factors associated with heart disease are hypertension, high cholesterol, diabetes, inadequate physical activity, cigarette smoking, and obesity. Lowering cholesterol levels and increasing the HDL—the good cholesterol—can be accomplished by diet alterations, increased physical activity, and losing excess

Table I.3
Age-Adjusted Cause of Death Rate per 100,000 for African American and White Females

Cause of Death	African American	White American
Heart disease	165.5	100.7
Cancer	136.3	111.2

Source: Horton, *Women's Health Data Book* (1995, adapted from table 3-1, p. 54).

weight. As previously mentioned, obesity continues to occur more often in African American women than in white women, it is imperative that controlling the "poverty diet," which is high in fats and sugar, becomes a priority. Also, psychological factors like racism, which causes stress and as the Farmingham study notes, stress does play a major role in women's coronary health (Maris, p. 73; Collins, 2003, p. 9).

Also, as shown in Table I.4, the incidence rate for cancer is somewhat higher for white women, (e.g. breast cancer) but the mortality rate is higher for Black women.

The economic impact of cancer in 2002 was $171 billion, plus another $60 billion for payments to physicians, hospitals, and for drugs (U.S. DHHS, 2003, p. 40). With so much money spent on just one illness, why do African American women do so poorly in America's health care system? Although one answer may be the racial disparities that exist in health care (e.g., access issues or no

Table I.4
Age-Adjusted Cancer Incidence per 100,000 and Mortality Rates for Women by Race, United States, 1990–1997

Sites	Incidence per 100,000 Women	
	White	Black
Breast	114.0	100.2
Lung & Bronchus	43.3	45.8
Colon/Rectum	36.6	45.2
Cervical	8.4	11.7
Endometrial/Uterine	22.5	15.0
	Mortality per 100,000 Women	
Breast	26.3	31.4
Lung/Bronchus	34.0	33.0
Colon/Rectum	14.3	19.9
Cervical	2.4	5.9
Endometrial/Uterine	3.1	5.8

Source: Horton, *The Women's Health Data Book* (1995, adapted from table 4-8, p. 76).

health insurance), this is not a new phenomenon. African Americans have had a poor start in their medical care since their first day on America's shores.

However, despite this disparity, African American women continue to survive, often triumphing despite disease. Some prominent survivors of breast cancer, for example, include Desiree Rogers, president of Peoples Gas and North Shore Gas; the Rev. Dr. Claudette Anderson Copeland, pastor and cofounder of the New Creation Christian Fellowship Church in San Antonio, Texas; and Marilyn Francine Braxton, controller of Chinagraphy and Darlene Nipper BET Foundation (Kinnon, 2004, p. 60). In reading the accounts of their bouts with cancer, I noticed some common themes: they recognized how stress adversely affect physical health, the importance of diet, physical activity and exercise, self breast examination, and faith, family, and friends.

Because of poor health outcomes for so many illnesses plaguing African American women, we must take charge of our health, as Copeland did when she demanded a biopsy of a lump in her breast. Now she shares her experience with breast cancer through her ministry (Kinnon, 2004, p. 64), using a health voice-message to help women to understand how important early detection and mamagrams are to their survival.

Alcohol use among African American women is another serious health behavioral problem. Alcohol each year accounts for over 100,000 deaths and billions in health care costs. Some have blamed the high divorce rate, 50 percent of family violence, and millions of hours of school and job absenteeism on alcohol abuse. Diseases and disorders associated with alcoholism, including cirrhosis, anemia, and fetal alcohol syndrome, are having a devastating impact on the African American female's health and her family relationships. Because most people believe they can drink and hold their liquor, uncontrollable drinking behavior is the contributing factor in this illness. In one study it was found that as many as 14 percent intoxicated college women engaged in unintended sexual activity (Mielman, 1993, p. 27). Women who are under the influence of drugs and alcohol may abandon the use of condoms and participate in unprotected sex, which increases their exposure to sexually transmitted diseases, including AIDS. Further:

Women who drink are more likely than men to develop liver cirrhosis and die from it.

Even three drinks a week increases the risk of breast cancer.

Drinking alcohol makes orgasm more difficult to achieve and lessens its intensity because its depresses the central nervous system.

Alcohol inhibits the body's ability to use vitamins and calcium. (Misra, 2000, p. 377)

Further, fetal alcohol syndrome, which is tied to birth defects from heavy drinking during pregnancy also paints a dismal picture of African American women drinking patterns. It was reported in The Women's Health Data Book (Horton, 1995) that "the incidence of fetal alcohol syndrome varies widely among different ethnic groups, ranging from 0.3 per 10,000 births for Asians, 0.8 for

Hispanics, 0.9 for whites, 6.0 for Blacks to a high of 29.9 for Native Americans (p. 106). When you combine alcohol use and illicit drug use (dual dependency), the effects are even more serious: "African American women are only 12.7% of America's female population and accounted for 26% of drug related deaths in 1999" (Leigh & Jimenez, 2003, p. 79). These women experience major risks from AIDS through injectable drugs, followed by heterosexual contact from un-protected sexual behavior, which includes unprotected intercourse with a person (e.g., boyfriend, husband) whom the women believe is committed to a hetero-sexual, monogamous relationship, but is actually having sex with other males—"being on the down low"—and ultimately spreading the AIDS virus.

In addition, an estimated 2 million prisoners are released each year into inner-city communities, further putting African American women at risk of exposure to STDs from males who have been exposed during their incarceration.

According to Misra (2000, p. 56) although the overall rate of new AIDS cases is decreasing, new cases are reported at a higher rate among Black women (75 per 100,000 population) as compared with whites (7 per 100,000). Four years later, African American women were reported to make up approximately 72 percent of new female cases of HIV (Carter, 2004, p. 99). As Donnie W. Watson, a clinical psychologist states, "Some minority researchers see substance abuse as a secondary problem, resulting from individual responses to primary problems of oppression, racism, economic deprivation, stress, and despair in society" (Braithwaite & Taylor, 1992, p. 64).

Some estimate that in America, on any given day, there are 4.6 million persons who suffer from some form of mental disorder, like depression. One illness that seems to be more pervasive in African American females is severe depression (DHHS, 2004, p. 24). Women make 2 million annual visits to mental health professionals (Collins, 2003, p. 16). Life crises, unemployment, sexism, poverty, high-stress jobs, single parenthood, and covert and overt racial discrimination make African American women particularly vulnerable to de-pression.

Another social ill that impacts the health status of African American women is poverty. According to Day (2003), the poverty rate of African American women was 22.1 percent in 2000, while the percentage for their counterparts was 9.4 (p. 15). In order to eliminate this disparity, a commitment is needed from the federal government, which, in the *National Healthcare Disparities Report* (DHHS, 2003), recognized that poverty is a critical determinant of health outcomes. This report also provided a "comprehensive view of the scope and characteristics of differences in health care quality and access as-sociated with patient race, ethnicity, income, education, and place of residence" (p. 37).

In this commentary several health and social problems that impact the health status of African American women were briefly presented to set the stage for a more in-depth discussion on the matter. It is up all who work in health care and set policy to do the right thing—to eradicate the social ills and health care disparity that so disproportionately affect African American women.

REFERENCES

Beardsley, E. 1990. Race as a Factor in Health. In *Women, Health and Medicine in America: A Historical Handbook*, Rima Apple, ed., pp. 121–140. New York: Garland.

Braithwaite, R., and S. Taylor. 1992. *Health Issues in the Black Community.* San Francisco: Jossey-Bass Publishers.

Carter, M. Z. 2004. Know Your State: The Latest News on HIV Testing Could Save Your Life. *Essence*, December, p. 99.

Collins, C. F. 1996. Commentary on The Health and Social Status of African American Women. In *African American Women's Health and Social Issues*, Catherine Collins, ed., pp. 1–10. Westport, Conn.: Praeger.

———. 2003. *Sources of Stress and Relief for African American Women.* Westport, Conn.: Praeger.

Day, P. 2003. *The New History of Social Welfare.* 4th ed. Boston, Mass.: Allyn & Bacon.

Delbanco, F. 2004. The Sexual Diseases Up to 75% of Young Women Will Get. *Glamour*, May, pp. 110–112.

Harper, A., and L. Lambert. 1994. *The Health of Populations: An Introduction.* 2nd ed. New York: Springer Publishing Company.

The State of Black Health Care in America. 2001. *HealthQuest* (Special Issue), June/July.

Hoffman, F. L. 1989. *Race, Traits and Tendencies of the American Negro.* New York: MacMillen Publishers.

Horton, A. J., ed. 1992. *The Women's Health Data Book: A Profile of Women's Health in the United States.* Washington, D.C.: The Jacobs Institute of Women's Health.

———. 1995. *The Women's Health Data Book: A Profile of Women's Health in the United States.* 2nd ed. Washington, D.C.: The Jacobs Institute of Women's Health.

Johnson, A. 2004–2005. How to Get More Health Professionals of Color, and Why It's a Life-and-Death Issue. *Diversity Inc.* December/January, p. 106.

Kinnon, B. J. 2004. I Survived Breast Cancer. *Ebony*, October, p. 60–67.

Leigh, W. 1994. *The Health Status of Women of Color.* A Women's Health Report of the Women's Research and Education Institute. Washington, D.C.: Women's Research and Education Institute.

Leigh, W., and M. Jimenez. 2003. *Women of Color Health Data Book.* Washington, D.C.: National Institute of Health. Office of the Director.

Meadows, A. 2004–2005. How to Get More Health Professionals of Color, and Why It's a Life-and-Death Issue. *Diversity Inc.* December/January, p. 105.

Mielman, P. 1993. Alcohol Induced Sexual Behavior on Campus. *Journal of American College Health* 42(1): 27–31.

Misra, Dawn. 2000. *The Women's Health Data Book.* Washington, D.C.: Jacobs Institute of Women's Health.

U.S. Center for Disease Control. 2001. National Center for Health Statistics. *Health United States, 2001, with Urban and Rural Health Chartbook*, (PHS) 2001–1232, p. 176, table 32. Hyattsville, Md.

U.S. Department of Health and Human Services. 2003. Agency for Healthcare Research and Quality, *National Healthcare Disparities Report.* Rockville, Md. July. Available online at www.qualitytools.ashr.gov/disparitiesreport.

———. 2004. *Women's Health in the U.S., Research on Health Issues Affecting Women.* National Institute of Health, National Institute of Allergy and Infectious Diseases. Hyattsville, Md.

Wallechinsky, D. 2005. Where Does Your Tax Money Go? *Buffalo News*, *Parade* magazine, April 10.

Wegman, E. M. 1990. Annual Summary of Vital Statistics 1989. *Pediatrics*, December, 8(6):841, Table 4.

———. 1993. Annual Summary of Vital Statistics 1992. *Pediatrics*, December, 92(6): 747, Table 4.

Weisman, J. 2003. U.S. Income Fell, Poverty Rose in 2002. *Washington Post*, September 27, p. 1.

1

African American Women
and Heart Disease

LYNNE VALENCIA PERRY-BOTTINGER, M.D.

Cardiovascular (heart) disease has been the leading cause of death for women and men of all ethnic groups in the United States since 1900 (except for influenza in 1918). Heart disease accounts for almost 40 percent of all deaths in this country and claims about as many lives each year as the next five leading causes of death combined (Figure 1.1). Heart disease kills about 10 times as many women as breast cancer.

According to the 2005 American Heart Association Statistics update, based on 2002 Centers for Disease Control (CDC) data, there are about 70 million people walking around with heart disease, and over half of those are women (American Heart Association, 2005). About 500,000 women die every year of cardiovascular disease, and a disproportionate number of those are African American women. Premature deaths, defined as the death of those younger than age 65, are 31.5 percent more likely for African Americans and 36 percent more for American Indians and Alaskan Natives (CDC, 2004).

Although the age-adjusted death rates for all heart disease have declined from 1990 to 1998, this is less so for the African American population. To give some perspective, take the Healthy People 2010 initiative, in which the federal government teamed up with major health organizations to reduce cardiovascular mortality by 25 percent. Since 1990, although it has declined 15 percent for whites, the death rate has declined only 11 percent for Blacks (Yancy et al., 2005).

First let us define what we mean by cardiovascular or heart disease. Basically, the heart is like a house. It has plumbing (the coronary arteries that sit on the outside of the heart), electricity (the conduction system that stimulates the heart muscle to pump), doors (the four valves, called tricuspid, pulmonic, mitral, and aortic, that help control blood flow from one chamber to the other), rooms (the

Figure 1.1
Leading Causes of Death for All Males and Females, United States: 2001

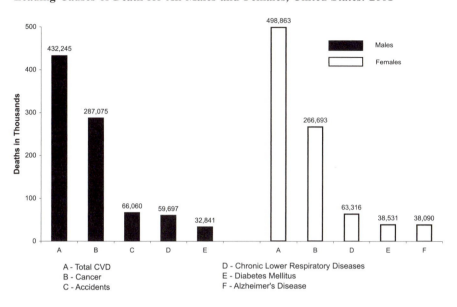

A - Total CVD
B - Cancer
C - Accidents

D - Chronic Lower Respiratory Diseases
E - Diabetes Mellitus
F - Alzheimer's Disease

four chambers, called right atrium, left atrium, right ventricle, and left ventricle, which hold blood).

The specialist who cares for the heart is a cardiologist. Most board-certified cardiologists can oversee all these areas, but if they need a little extra attention, a cardiology subspecialist such as an interventional cardiologist or cardiac surgeon (plumber), electrophysiologist (electrician), or cardiomyopathy expert (heart muscle specialist) may be required.

TYPES OF HEART DISEASE

There are six basic different types of heart disease that affect most adults. The major type is coronary heart disease (CHD; also called coronary artery disease) which affects 13 million people, of whom about 6 million are women. This refers to blockages in the blood vessels that feed blood to the heart. Significant blockages in these arteries cause heart attack or death of heart muscle (doctors call this acute coronary syndrome or myocardial infarction), potentially fatal irregular heart rhythms (doctors call this supraventricular or ventricular tachycardia), or fluid backup in the lungs (doctors call this heart failure and in the past used the term congestive heart failure) (Figure 1.2).

Be aware that the first sign of CHD may be sudden death. About 50 percent of men and 64 percent of women who died suddenly of CHD had no previous symptoms of the disease, according to National Heart, Lung, and Blood Institute (NHLBI) data compiled by Dr. J. Willis Hurst (American Heart Association, 2005). There are about 1.2 million heart attacks annually in this country, and

Figure 1.2
Coronary Artery Disease

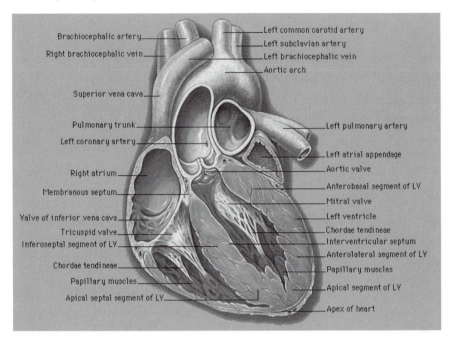

most of them are first heart attacks. Women are more likely to die, to become disabled, and to have a second heart attack than men are. African American women are most likely to die.

The second type of cardiovascular disease is hypertension or high blood pressure, which affects all of the major arteries of the body, including those in the heart. The increased stress on the heart causes the main pumping chamber, called the left ventricle, to thicken and enlarge over time. Doctors call this left ventricular hypertrophy (LVH). The oldest population study on heart disease in this country was called the Framingham study. It found that the presence of LVH is one of the greatest predictors of a patient dying a cardiovascular death (Levy et al., 1990). Hypertension is defined as blood pressure equal to or greater than 140/90 on at least two seated occasions or taking antihypertensive medication, according to the seventh report of the Joint National Committee on Prevention, Detection, Evaluation, and Treatment of High Blood Pressure. This committee also designated a new category, called prehypertension, and Stage 2 and 3 hypertension were combined (Chobanian et al., 2003) (Figure 1.3). Hypertension affects 65 million people in the United States.

About 59 million people have prehypertension, which refers to systolic blood pressure (the top number) of 120–139 and diastolic blood pressure of 80–89. These people are at high risk of developing hypertension and its complications. Patients and physicians should aim for ideal blood pressure of 120/80 in all

Figure 1.3
Hypertension Guidelines

JNC VII-Seventh Report of the Joint National Committee on Prevention, Detection, Evaluation, and Treatment of High Blood Pressure

- Pre-htn: **SBP 120-139 or DBP 80-89**
- Stage I htn: **SBP 140-159 or DBP 90-99**
- Stage II htn: **SBP $\geq$ 160 or DBP $\geq$ 100**

(Chobanian et al., *JAMA*, 289:2560-72, 2003)

Note: htn = hypertension; SBP = systolic blood pressure; DBP = diastolic blood pressure.

Source: Chobanian et al., 2003.

patients and perform a basic diagnostic workup with complete eye, cardiovascular, pulmonary, and abdominal exam; electrocardiogram; serum chemistries; complete blood count; urinalysis; and consideration for echocardiogram or sonogram of the heart. This applies particularly to the diabetic patient, for whom the committee criteria for acceptable blood pressure have been tightened from 130/80 to 120/80.

There are a myriad of causes of systemic hypertension, but most of the cases affecting African Americans as well as other patients are essential or idiopathic hypertension. Other causes include renal or kidney disease; autoimmune disease like systemic lupus erythematosus; endocrine or hormonal diseases like pheochromocytoma or Graves disease (hyperthyroidism); head injury; substance abuse with alcohol, cocaine, or amphetamines; or nonsteroidal antiinflammatory drugs such as ibuprofen. Hypertension can be brought on by severe mental or physical stress such as weightlifting or pregnancy.

African Americans appear to have the highest prevalence of hypertension in the world. Although about a third of the Caucasian American and European populations have hypertension, according to the National Health and Nutrition Survey Data for 1999–2002, about 45 percent of African American women and 42 percent of African American men over the age of 20 have high blood pressure. For years cardiologists like Dr. Elijah Saunders, Dr. Julian Haywood, and Dr. Keith Ferdinand have stated that African Americans develop high blood pressure earlier in life and more severely than their Caucasian counterparts (Saunders, 1991). Physiologists, like Dr. Friedrich Luft in 1977, demonstrated that one reason may be that young African Americans have less suppression of plasma renin activity (Luft et al., 1979). Renin is an important hormone involved in sodium or salt regulation in the body, and many blood pressure medicines work by controlling its activity. If one cannot suppress renin, one is more likely to retain salt, and as a result, one is more likely to retain water.

When I practiced medicine in southern Africa for a few months in the 1990s, I did not see the degree of hypertension or the ravages of its complications that I have seen in the United States. Reasons as to why African Americans in the

United States have the highest prevalence range from repeated social stresses such as racism and poverty to a high sodium/high fat diet to genetic influences. For example, as Dr. Clyde Yancy summarizes in a recent issue dedicated to cardiovascular ethnic disparities in *Circulation,* variability in genes located on chromosome 4 that control mineralocorticoid function may explain early-onset hypertension in African Americans. Another possible gene culprit is the C825T polymorphism of the gene encoding for the G protein B3 subunit, which may confer a greater risk of left ventricular hypertrophy. These appear to be more common in African Americans, Africans, and Aborigines (Yancy et al., 2005). Meanwhile we must not forget how dangerous anger can be. Dr. Patrick Steffen found that African Americans who said they often held back feelings of anger tended to show a smaller drop in blood pressure than normally occurs during bedtime (Steffen et al., 2003).

Deaths occur from end organ damage from the effects of elevated blood pressure and include eye damage including blindness, stroke, kidney failure, and heart failure. In addition, hypertension is an independent risk factor for coronary heart disease and can make diabetes all the more difficult to treat. Dr. William Parmley, former president of the American College of Cardiology, summarized in a call-to-action editorial in that association's journal that African Americans are 350 percent more likely to die from hypertension than Caucasians, 80 percent more likely to die from stroke, 320 percent more likely to get kidney failure, and 150 percent more likely to die from heart failure. African Americans are 6 times more likely to die from end-stage kidney disease for a variety of reasons. These include late disease detection, lack of access to care, and reduced referral for kidney transplantation (Parmley, 2004).

The third type of cardiovascular disease is valvular heart disease, which means a leak or blockage in one of the four valves that control blood flow in the heart. Although overall this disease is in decline, it is most dangerous for women during pregnancy and old age. The exception is mitral valve prolapse—a common condition in women that presents in young adulthood, is usually benign, and is of little clinical significance. This refers to a "floppy heart valve" or click phenomenon. It is estimated that up to 1 percent of women have mitral valve prolapse. If you refer to the heart diagram you will see the mitral valve helps connect the left atrium and left ventricle. The one situation that may pose a problem for mitral valve patients is when the valve "leaks" (i.e., blood flows back through the door when it should be closed). If the leak is severe, blood can back up into the lungs, creating the condition called heart failure. Patients may get short of breath in this case. To prevent this and any infection that could lead to it (known as endocarditis), patients who already have a leak are asked to take an antibiotic before dental procedures or gastrointestinal or genitourinary procedures. If infection has already set in, it is important to get prompt intravenous antibiotic therapy. Sometimes patients may get a leak even without an infection. The dangerous type of valvular heart disease for the pregnant patient is one that creates or worsens pulmonary hypertension or high blood pressure in the lungs. (This is not to be confused with systemic hypertension, as described previously.) The problem with pulmonary hypertension and the pregnant woman is that it becomes all the more difficult for the woman herself to get enough oxygen, thereby putting her and the fetus at high risk of death. The common type of heart disease seen in the elderly is aortic valve disease. The aortic valve may leak (usually called aortic insufficiency) or close off (aortic stenosis). Usually the latter is a more serious problem and requires surgical consideration if the patient is passing out, experiencing chest pain, or getting short of breath. Aortic insufficiency is usually due to high blood pressure and can be managed medically unless the patient is developing symptoms of severe shortness of breath or leg swelling or has a complicating issue like aortic dissection/aneurysm (tear or bulging of the great blood vessel that carries blood throughout the body) or infection of the valve. Both of these situations usually require surgical repair of the valve.

The fourth type is arrhythmia or abnormal heart rhythm, which can be a result of any of the previous problems or occur on its own and can also be fatal. It affects almost a million Americans annually (American Heart Association, 2005). Normally the heart has its own pacemaker, called the sinoatrial node and located at the top of the heart. When stimulated, it sends signals throughout the top part of the heart, which meet at the atrioventricular node and then proceed through each of the two ventricles. If one or more of these electrical impulses shortcircuits at the top, that can create a situation called heart block, where impulses cannot reach the bottom chambers properly. If there are too many electrical impulses at the top of the heart, that creates a situation called supraventricular tachycardia. The top part of the heart beats very quickly and at times the bottom part of the heart cannot keep up, and so some of the impulses will be blocked. If there are too many electrical impulses being generated by the bottom of the heart, that creates an even more dangerous situation called ventricular tachycardia. In either case, the heart beats too quickly, the patient may get a sensation of the heart pounding or racing, pressure, shortness of breath, and dizziness, or may actually pass out. The reason ventricular tachycardia is more dangerous is there is virtually no way for the heart to block the rapid impulses that generate there, and this rhythm can degenerate in ventricular fibrillation, which can cause sudden cardiac death. These problems can usually be repaired by finding the underlying problem, giving medications to control the heart rhythm, or inserting a pacemaker (or in the case of ventricular tachycardia/fibrillation, a defibrillator). I recommend the families of patients with the most dangerous types of rhythms learn cardiopulmonary resuscitation (CPR) taught by the American Heart Association and consider investing in a defibrillator for the home.

Heart failure or heart muscle problem (also called cardiomyopathy), the fifth type, is increasing in incidence and affects 5 million people with about 550,000 new cases each year (American Heart Association, 2005). Heart failure refers to the failure of the heart—specifically the left ventricle—to function as a pump. Sudden death is responsible for more than 50 percent of the mortality from this disease. It is more common in the elderly, particularly the African American elderly. Again, heart failure can occur as a result of hypertension or coronary artery, valvular, or arrhythmia disease, but it can also arise on its own. When heart failure appears to arise on its own, it is important to rule out toxins such as alcohol, cocaine, amphetamines, or some prescription drugs; infections such as human immunodeficiency virus (HIV) or trypanosomiasis; autoimmune disease; and unusual illnesses such as sarcoidosis or amyloidosis; as well as familial etiologies such as idiopathic hypertrophic subaortic stenosis. While some athletes who die suddenly performing a sport may bring attention to the importance of screening for cardiomyopathy, these cases are relatively rare. By far the biggest proportion is from poorly treated hypertension.

The sixth type of cardiovascular disease is stroke or severe impairment of blood flow to the head. This affects 5.4 million people in the United States and slightly more women than men. Of the 700,000 new and recurrent strokes each year, 53 percent occur in women and disproportionately in African American women. According to the American Heart Association, whereas every 26 seconds an American has a coronary artery event, every 45 seconds an American has a stroke. Stroke in itself is the third leading cause of death in this country and a leading cause of disability (American Heart Association, 2005). The Southeast (particularly North and South Carolina and Georgia) has the highest stroke incidence according to the CDC's 2003 *Atlas of Stroke Mortality*. Jacobs reported in the Northern Manhattan Stroke Study of 2003 that even young (age 20–44) Black and Hispanic women and men are 2.4 times as likely as whites to suffer stroke. That difference in incidence increases through middle age to up to 5 times as likely, but the racial difference declines after age 65 (Jacobs et al., 2002). The Reasons for Geographic and Racial Differences Study (REGARDS) tried to define why these differences exist. Unfortunately, the CDC reported in January 2005 that the stroke mortality gap continues to widen (American Heart Association, 2005). In the same report, African Americans and women said to be more likely to be admitted to a skilled nursing facility rather than go home after their stroke hospitalization than their Caucasian male counterparts. The major stroke symptoms are weakness or numbness of the face, arm, and leg on one side of the body; sudden dizziness; loss of vision; unsteadiness; falls; headache; loss of speech; and difficulty speaking.

A rarer type of heart disease, which is rarely deadly is pericarditis. This condition refers to inflammation around the lining of the heart. The pain it produces may be severe and mimic a heart attack but is usually worse on inspiration. Pericarditis can be diagnosed by electrocardiogram (ECG or EKG). If diagnosed, it is important to get an echocardiogram or ultrasound test of the heart to make sure there is no buildup of fluid around the heart (known as an effusion). In severe cases, this is called cardiac tamponade and can be serious, since it may restrict blood from entering the heart and needs to be drained with a needle. Pericarditis is usually caused by a virus, kidney failure, autoimmune disease, or cancer.

Coronary heart disease remains the leading cause of death for both sexes in the United States, and the overall prevalence in this country is estimated at 12 million people. It affects 3 million women and 4.2 million men. Ten times as many women die of coronary heart disease as die from breast cancer (Figure 1.4). African American women and men have higher mortality from all types of heart disease than Caucasians and are 40 percent more likely to die from heart disease. In fact *heart disease kills 41 percent of all African American women,* according

Figure 1.4
Percentage Breakdown of Deaths from Cardiovascular Diseases, United States, 2001

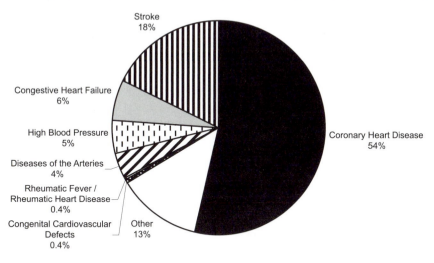

to the Centers for Disease Control (CDC, 2004). Since coronary heart disease is overwhelmingly responsible for most American deaths, I will direct most of my attention to this problem.

Both women and physicians underestimate the impact of the severity of heart disease on women. According to an American Heart Association survey of 1,024 women (with oversampling of African American and Hispanic women) reported in 2004, almost half of women realized heart attack was the leading killer of women (up from about 30 percent of women in 2000). Drs. Lori Mosca and Anjanette Ferris found that white women were more informed than Black and Hispanic women on early treatments available for heart attack victims. In the same study, significantly more Caucasian women than African Americans or Hispanics discussed heart disease with their doctor. Overall only 38 percent of women actually discussed heart disease at all with their physician (Mosca et al., 2004b).

HEART DISEASE RISK FACTORS

The major coronary heart disease risk factors are hypertension, diabetes, abnormal cholesterol profile, obesity, tobacco use, and premature family history (first heart attack in a male first-degree relative under age 55 or female first-degree relative less than age 65). Diabetes and obesity also are disproportionately high in the African American population. In the Atherosclerosis Risk in Communities (ARIC) study, African American women had a 2.4-fold greater incidence of type 2 diabetes than their Caucasian counterparts. Type 2 diabetes in American adults is frequently associated with the metabolic (also known as dysmetabolic) syndrome, which comprises obesity, insulin resistance, hypertension, and proinflammatory/prothrombotic state. (*Proinflammatory/prothrombotic* refers to the tendency to build up clot on top of cholesterol plaques). Yet Dr. Karol Watson reports that African Americans have a higher prevalence of resistance to insulin even after controlling for obesity and lifestyle factors (Watson, 2005). Women who are diabetic are 3 to 7 times more likely to have heart disease, whereas men who are diabetic are only 2 to 4 times more likely (Rich-Edwards et al., 1995). According to the CDC, diabetes in increasing, particularly in the minority population. African Americans and Hispanics have higher rates of diabetes, independent of weight, with rates almost tripling in the past 30 years. They have twice the rate of whites (American Heart Association, 2005). The National Cholesterol Education panel's third report defined diabetes as risk equivalent to coronary heart disease. That is, people who have diabetes should have their cholesterol profiles managed as aggressively as those who already have coronary heart disease (National Cholesterol Education Program, 2001).

Abnormal cholesterol profile does not just mean having a high total cholesterol, as it once did. It means having an elevated level of low-density lipoprotein (LDL) or a low level of high-density lipoprotein (HDL). Remember LDL is "lousy" or bad cholesterol and HDL is good cholesterol. Although African Americans do not have as many cholesterol abnormalities as Caucasians, Dr. Alan Gould reported that 41.6 percent of African American women and 46.3 percent of African American men older than 20 have markedly abnormal levels of bad cholesterol (Gould et al., 1998) (Figure 1.5). It is the bad cholesterol that clogs the arteries to create the blockages that cause heart attacks. Young, healthy African Americans generally have a better cholesterol profile than their Caucasian counterparts. "Better" means 10–20 percent higher levels of HDL, or good, cholesterol, according to Dr. Karol Watson (2005). HDL is cardioprotective primarily because it helps transport cholesterol through the body and inhibits plaque growth.

For people who already have heart disease or diabetes mellitus, the LDL level should be 70 or less. For those patients with two risk factors and thus at moderate risk, the LDL cholesterol should be less than 100 (Grundy et al., 2004). For those at low risk, LDL values of 130–160 are tolerated (National Cholesterol Education Program, 2001). The optimal HDL level for women is 50 or more (40 for men) (Ashen et al., 2005). Women should be aware that HDL may decline with age, smoking, or sedentary lifestyle.

Before menopause, women are less likely than men to have coronary heart disease unless they have diabetes, hypertension, or family history. After menopause (especially 10–15 years out), women have similar risk of heart disease and subsequent death as men and 2 to 3 times the risk of premenopausal women (American Heart Association, 2005).

Forget the ideal weight charts. Obesity is now defined as body mass index (BMI) over 30. BMI takes the height into account. It is calculated as weight (in pounds) × 703 ÷ height × height (in inches) or weight (in kilograms) ÷ height × height (in meters). It should be taken seriously when greater than 25 because then you are overweight and on the way to be obese. In the Nurses' Health Study, a cohort of 115,886 predominantly Caucasian women aged 30–55, started in 1976 and continued for years, obesity was associated with a threefold

Figure 1.5
Percentages of Americans > 20 with LDL-C Levels ≥ 130

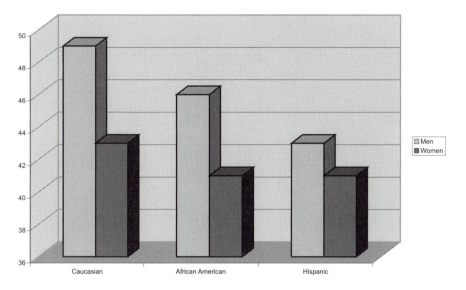

increase in coronary heart disease deaths. Dr. Joann Manson also reported that even overweight women in the 25–29 BMI or Quetlet range had increased coronary heart disease incidence (Manson et al., 1990). Body mass index has been criticized as perhaps not being as reliable in the African American patient. Dr. Lori Mosca and others report that the waist size is also a useful predictor of coronary heart disease event rates. Women should have a waist size less than 35 inches (Mosca et al., 2004a).

African Americans have the highest prevalence of obesity in the United States of any ethnic group. Overall the incidence of obesity is slightly over 30 percent. Moreover, 77 percent of Black women are overweight and almost 50 percent are obese. A similar number of Hispanic women are overweight and obese (Figure 1.6). Obesity kills 300,000 people yearly and is the second most preventable cause of heart disease (American Heart Association, 2005).

There are also several emerging risk factors: C-reactive protein, homocysteine, lipoprotein (a), interleukin 6, and serum amyloid A. The search for other cardiovascular markers began when Dr. Eugene Braunwald reported in 1997 that half of all heart attacks occur in people with normal lipid levels (Braunwald, 1997). Based on the recognition that atherosclerosis or plaque buildup is an inflammatory process, several plasma markers were evaluated (Ross, 1999). Dr. Paul Ridker evaluated C-reactive protein and other plasma marker levels in the 28,263 women in the Nurses' Health Study and found the strongest association between elevated high-sensitivity C-reactive protein and cardiovascular events (Ridker et al., 2000). African American women appear to have the highest C-reactive protein levels among women (Mensah et al., 2005). This is usually treated by treating the traditional cardiovascular risk factors and with statin therapy (to be

Figure 1.6
Prevalence of Obesity (BMI > 31), Adults 20–80

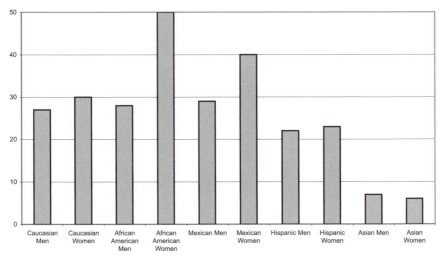

Note: Dem = demographic.

Source: Centers for Disease Control, 2004.

discussed later). The association between elevated homocysteine and cardio-vascular events such as heart attack was first described in Caucasian men but is found in African American women also. This is usually treated by folate therapy since this has been found to reduce plaque buildup (Schnyder et al., 2001).

HEART ATTACK

There are 1.2 million heart attack patients a year, and 60 percent of these patients are women (American Heart Association, 2005). Heart attacks are caused by arteries with some degree of plaque buildup or atherosclerosis becoming completely blocked by a blood clot or pieces of the plaque being released and clogging the blood vessel downstream. This complete cessation of blood flow causes the death of heart muscle. Doctors refer to this as myocardial infarction or acute coronary syndrome (Figure 1.7). Most patients die before coming to the hospital from arrhythmia or irregular heart rhythm created by toxic buildup of dying muscle.

The classic heart attack symptom is crushing chest pain on exertion. During a heart attack, women are more likely than men to have non–chest-related symptoms. In addition to sustained chest pain, pressure, and a feeling of fullness, either with or without exertion, women also have shortness of breath, nausea, vomiting, sweating, palpitations, fatigue, and jaw, neck, abdominal, shoulder, arm, or back pain.

These symptoms may be elusive in the African American women, but in my practice I have found sudden onset of poor blood pressure control a strong clue.

Figure 1.7
Features of a Ruptured Atherosclerotic Plaque

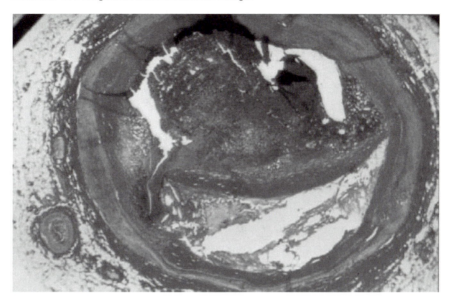

In her book, *Sources of Stress and Relief for African American Women,* Dr. Catherine Collins gives the sister's perspective on having a heart attack.

Over long periods of stress, our heart which normally beats 100,000 times a day, speeds up, sending blood rushing through our veins and arteries.... When African American women encounter a stressful situation (such as racism), their heart rate increases and some of these fatty deposits may become dislodged and freely float until they reach a location where they are stopped. This causes a decrease in blood flow to the heart and makes the heart work harder. Over long periods when black women face a constant barrage of unpleasant events, the heart races and pumps harder because of the clogged blood vessels decreasing the flow of blood. (Collins, 2003, p. 8)

The only way to know you are having a heart attack is to get to the hospital and get an electrocardiogram and a blood test called cardiac troponin or, in the past, creatine phospokinase (CPK-MB). These are highly sensitive markers for heart attacks. Do not leave the emergency room without them.

GENDER AND ETHNIC DISPARITIES

There are cases of patients being sent home while having a heart attack. One study found the likelihood of this happening is highest if the patient is an African American woman. Nonwhite women younger than age 55 are the most likely patients to be sent home from the emergency room (Pope et al., 2000).

During a heart attack, women are more likely to die (African American women are twice as likely) than men (Keil et al., 1993). Women are more likely to be disabled, more likely to have another heart attack, more likely to develop heart failure and heart rupture (Wenger et al., 1993; Petrie, 1999; Hochman et al., 1999). Women are less likely to be referred for life-saving treatments and for cardiac rehabilitation (Ades, 2001; Healy, 1990). Part of this is that women are older and have more illnesses than men when they have their first heart attack—but only a small part.

Dr. Cynthia Crawford-Green pointed to many of the reasons in the 1996 edition of *African American Women's Health and Social Issues*. They are: lack of access to a health care provider, inability to afford medications, intolerable side effects of medications, lack of close follow-up by the treating physician, and inattention to inadequately controlled blood pressure, obesity, smoking, and stress (Crawford-Green, 1996).

Despite a higher mortality, African American women have a lower prevalence of obstructive coronary disease than their Caucasian or Asian counterparts (Budoff et al., 2002). African Americans in the Multi-Ethnic Study of Atherosclerosis (MESA) study also had lower incidence of coronary calcification (Bild et al., 2005). In some patients, coronary calcification is a marker of atherosclerotic plaque and predictive of coronary events. This does not appear to be always true in African Americans. This is important because newer scans, such as high-resolution computed tomography, used to detect the degree of coronary calcification may not be as predictive in the African American patient.

Summarizing several studies that discussed the female bias in cardiac testing, Dr. Bernadine Healy, first female director of the National Institutes of Health, coined the term *Yentl syndrome* in her editorial in the *New England Journal of Medicine* in 1990, where several major trials showing bias in cardiac care were presented. Women were referred less for advanced cardiac testing prior to having a heart attack, but when they presented with a heart attack in the manner a man would, they were treated appropriately and referred for advanced cardiac testing (Healy, 1990). Recognizing the bias was critical because the issue of women's lack of involvement in clinical trials was addressed. In 1993 the National Institutes of Health (NIH) issued guidelines for the inclusion of women as subjects in clinical trials, mandating that the intervention or therapy being studied must be evaluated as to whether it affects women differently (NIH, 1994). Nevertheless, in a study looking at the number of women involved in the 593 coronary heart disease trials, female enrollment rose from only 20 percent from 1966–1990 to 25 percent from 1991–2000 (Lee et al., 2001).

The key question about having a heart attack caused by a blocked artery is how fast the artery can be opened. Doctors use the term *reperfusion* to refer to restoring blood flow to the artery. Heart attack victims should immediately be considered for a medication called fibrinolytic or thrombolytic (clotbuster) or a procedure to look at and open the arteries, procedures called *cardiac catheterization* and *percutaneous coronary intervention* (coronary angioplasty), respectively (Figures 1.8 and 1.9). Basically, if angioplasty is available at the hospital or the patient can be transferred to a hospital to have the procedure done as soon as possible, many cardiologists will choose this approach. For most heart attacks in women, Dr. Alexandra Lansky, who headed a 2005 American Heart Association

Figure 1.8
Cardiac Catheterization

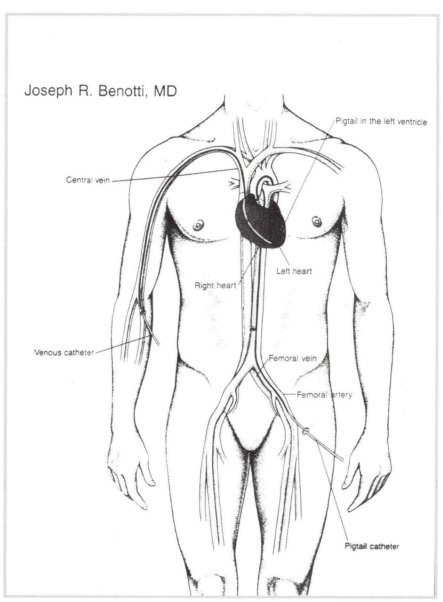

committee convened to define angioplasty guidelines for women, recommends angioplasty as the preferred alternative (Lansky et al., 2005). Nevertheless, doctors continue to underutilize these measures for African American women.

A commonly cited study is Dr. Schulman's research, reported in the *New England Journal of Medicine* in 1999, on the effect of race and sex on 720

Figure 1.9
Percutaneous Coronary Intervention

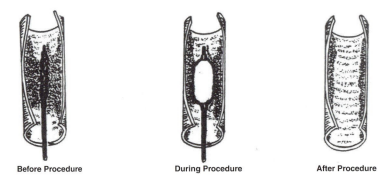

Before Procedure   During Procedure   After Procedure

primary care physicians. This included physicians' (30 percent female) recommendations for cardiac catheterization. These physicians evaluated eight actors from different demographic groups (predominantly Caucasian and African American) who had the same scripted case histories of chest pain, insurance, and occupations. Women and minorities were referred at one half the rate white men were. African American women were referred the least (Schulman, 1999). This study can be criticized because it involved actors, however.

In the real world, we see much of the same. There have been numerous studies about the racial difference in referral for invasive cardiac procedures to repair the arteries in coronary heart disease patients. Since 1990, numerous studies from around the country have shown African Americans are referred less for diagnostic procedures and treatments to repair the coronary arteries than Caucasian patients. In fact, the Kaiser Family and American College of Cardiology Foundations presented a literature review to all of their members, which stated that from 1984 to 2001, 68 of 81 studies found racial and ethnic differences in cardiac care. The differences persisted despite controlling for age, amount of other illnesses, and socioeconomic status as defined by insurance ("Racial/Ethnic Differences," 2002). One theory to explain the disparity was that perhaps these cardiac procedures were overused in the Caucasian population. One interesting study looking at 4000 Caucasian and African American Medicare beneficiaries found that African Americans are referred for these procedures 1.7 times less even when accounting for the inappropriate overuse in Caucasian patients (Schneider et al., 2001). Another study summarizing findings from the CRUSADE (acronym for Can Rapid Risk Stratification of Unstable Angina Patients Suppress Adverse Outcomes with Early Implementation of the American College of Cardiology/ American Heart Association guidelines) study showed that the 5504 African American patients were less likely than 37,813 Caucasians to receive many of the evidence-based treatments. This included medications as well as procedures (Sonel et al., 2005). The most recent disparity follow-up study from 2005 looking at all Medicare beneficiaries from 1992–2001 (about 29 million people) found that disparities heart surgery worsened in most hospital regions, improved in a few, and that no national or local effort was taken to eliminate the racial disparities (Jha et al., 2005).

CARDIAC PROCEDURES

The usual methods of cardiac evaluation are electrocardiogram, echocardiogram, stress testing, and newer methods like positron emission tomography (PET), magnetic resonance imaging (MRI), and high resolution computed tomography (SPECT MPI). Dr. Jennifer Mieres describes the best stress testing techniques for the moderate risk patient in her 2005 review in Cardiology Special Section. The low energy radioactive tracer isotope thallium in most labs has been replaced by higher energy technetium-based agents such as cardiolite (Mieres et al., 2005). Stress testing is usually done with a physician and technologist in attendance monitoring a patient either walking, biking, or being injected with medications such as dobutamine, adenosine, or dipyridamole with electrocardiograms taken before, during, and after, and imaging done before and after exercise.

The high risk patient frequently required advanced cardiac testing. This implies more than the usual noninvasive methods of evaluating the heart such as stress testing with electrocardiograms, echocardiograms, or radioactive tracers but actually invasive diagnostic testing called cardiac catheterization. Cardiac catheterization remains the gold standard for determining severity of coronary artery disease and the required preliminary step for coronary revascularization or repairing the arteries. Cardiac catheterization and percutaneous transluminal coronary angioplasty and coronary artery bypass surgery are safer than in the past. Patients of all ages get these procedures all over the world. Cardiac cath is performed through a needle puncture in the groin or the forearm. A tube is advanced to the heart through the aorta. The aorta is the big blood vessel in the center of the body which resembles a tree trunk. The arteries to the body's various organs are like branches of the tree. A syringe of dye outside of the body is injected into the tube to show all of the arteries in the heart. It usually lasts less than an hour and patients go home the same day unless there is some severe abnormality.

Other than heart attack, the major indications for cardiac catheterization with suspected or known coronary disease are severe cardiac symptoms with minimal exertion or at rest while taking medical treatment, patients who have successfully been resuscitated from sudden cardiac death or have sustained ventricular tachycardia (dangerous frequently lethal heart rhythm disturbance) (American College of Cardiology, 2005).

The arteries are repaired through percutaneous coronary intervention also called percutaneous coronary transluminal coronary angioplasty or coronary artery bypass graft surgery. Percutaneous transluminal coronary angioplasty just means that a balloon is put into the tube as it is advanced to the heart to open the arteries. To make sure the result stays great, most doctors now place a stent over the newly opened area. The stent is a wire device that looks like the coil in a ballpoint pen and stays in the heart forever. Sometimes they close off. To prevent that, doctors now sometimes use a medicine surrounding the stent to keep it open. These are called drug-eluting stents. They have reduced the rates of stent restenosis in half (Moses et al., 2003). Doctors also give blood thinners before, during, and for at least a year after the procedure to keep the result looking good. Patients stay in the hospital overnight. The blockages can recur suddenly if the medicines are stopped.

If coronary heart disease is extensive, coronary artery bypass surgery is required. This is an invasive procedure that requires opening the chest and taking veins from the leg or arteries from the chest and inserting them across the blocked artery and sewing the other side directly to the aorta to restore blood flow. Patients stay in the hospital several days.

Studies have shown that when controlling for preexisting illnesses, African Americans did as well as Caucasians up to 12 years out from coronary artery bypass grafting. Being a Medicaid patient (which most African American patients were) hampered long-term survival (Zacharias et al., 2005).

If the heart has already sustained severe damage and is weak, placement of a left ventricular assist device (LVAD) or heart transplantation where a beating heart is taken from a brain-dead donor may be required (Rose et al., 2001). The heart is then transplanted into a waiting recipient. Heart transplantation takes many hours and patients usually are carefully prescreened and remain hospitalized for weeks. They are then followed closely to see if they "reject" the heart. This means the body mounts a large immune response against the donated tissue and requires immunosuppressant therapy and in rare cases a new heart to save the patient's life.

About 1.5 million cardiac catheterizations, 657,000 angioplasties, 515,000 coronary artery bypass graft surgeries, and 2,057 heart transplants were performed annually in 2002 in the United States according to the American Heart Association (2004).

There is also a racial discrepancy in receiving life-saving stroke treatment. In one 1999 study, even among the small subset of 189 good candidates, whites were 3 times more likely than blacks to get a clot buster (Johnston, 2001).

CARDIAC MEDICAL THERAPY

For both women and men of all ethnicities who have suffered a heart attack or myocardial infarction, beta blockers, angiotensin converting enzyme (ace) inhibitors, angiotensin II antagonists, aspirin, and blood thinners called heparin, clopidogrel, and glycoprotein IIBIIIA inhibitors, aldosterone antagonists have been proven in multiple trials to decrease the incidence of subsequent cardiac events (Mosca et al., 2004a). This is called secondary prevention. In the guidelines for heart disease prevention in women, patients are stratified by their risks, as described in Figure 1.10.

Still African American women get referred less for lifesaving measures than Caucasian women. For example, in the Heart and Estrogen Progestin trial of hormone replacement summarized later in this chapter, African American women were less likely to receive aspirin or statins, despite double the coronary heart disease event rate (Jha et al., 2003).

Figure 1.10
ACC/AHA Guidelines for CHD Prevention in Women—Risk Groups

ACC/AHA Guidelines for CHD Prevention in Women-Risk Groups

- High > 20%-known CHD/PVD/stroke/DM/ renal dz
- Intermediate 10-20%-subclincal CVD, metabolic syndrome, multiple risks, family hx
- Low < 10%-1 or no risks

Mosoa et al., *JACC* 2004; 43:000-21.

Source: Mosca et al., 2004a.

If you have any of the heart attack or stroke symptoms listed here, ask your doctor now if it would be okay for you to chew two regular strength 325 mg aspirin, as this may save your life. Take them, and call 911 without delay. Do not drive or have someone drive you to the emergency room. Ask your doctor first, since aspirin can cause significant gastrointestinal distress. Do not take acetaminophen or nonsteroidal antiinflammatory agents in this situation, as they are ineffective. Do not take cyclooxygenase 2 inhibitors, as some have been associated with increased heart attack risk (Graham et al., 2005).

The medicines used to treat high cholesterol are the bile acid sequestrants, fibric acid derivatives, niacin, small intestine brush border enzyme inhibitors (ezetimibe), statins (h-methoxyglutaryl reductase inhibitors), or a combination of these. The most effective are the statins, which also happen to be the most feared due to rare risks of liver inflammation or muscle weakness or destruction. They have side effects, but remember the likelihood is much lower than that of dying from the effects of high cholesterol. Lowering cholesterol reduces death rates from heart disease in all patients, irrespective of ethnicity, gender, and age. (See Figure 1.11 for acronyms for the largest trials, plus starting levels of LDL cholesterol).

There are now hundreds of drugs being used to treat hypertension. The major goal is to prevent damage to the brain, kidney, heart, and eyes. Drug types include diuretics, beta blockers, calcium channel blockers, aldosterone antagonists, ace inhibitors, and angiotensin receptor antagonists. For the African American patient, I refer to the consensus statement of the Hypertension in African Americans Working Group led by Dr. Janice Douglas (Douglas et al., 2003). I aim for target blood pressure of 120/80. I consider starting with a thiazide-type diuretic if feasible, but I am very likely to start a multidrug regimen. I also reinforce the adjunctive measures listed in the next section.

The conventional therapies for heart failure include diuretics, ace inhibitors, angiotensin receptor antagonists, aldosterone antagonists, vasodilators such as hydralazine, and beta blockers such as carvedilol. Digoxin is no longer commonly used for heart failure alone. For the African American patient with severe heart failure, a new drug called Bidil has been approved by the U.S. Food and Drug Administration (FDA). Based on previous trials suggesting Black patients have a clinically significant response to a combination of isosorbide dinitrate and

Figure 1.11
Secondary Coronary Artery Disease Prevention in Women

Study/Year	LDL	↓Mortality
■ 49 (Simvastatin) 1994	188	30%
■ CARE (Pravastatin) 1998	139	24%
■ LIPID (Pravastatin) 1998	150	22%
■ AVERT (Atorvastat.) 1999	115	36%
■ MIRACL (Ator.80) 2001	124	16%
■ Heart Protect(Simvastatin) 2002	131	24%
■ PROSPER (Prav40)2002	130	2.1%
■ PROVE-IT(Ator vs. Prav) 2004	106	16%

hydralazine, Dr. Anne Taylor and colleagues conducted a randomized trial of 1,050 self-described Black patients. Despite the controversy that ensued over whether to approve a drug for a specific race, the study demonstrated a 43 percent reduction in the death rate from any cause. The theory is that Blacks appear to have a lower availability of nitric oxide, which this drug helps provide (Taylor et al., 2004).

CARDIOVASCULAR PREVENTION

I tell patients that the best way to avoid having me become their personal plumber to clean their arteries is to conduct a little preventative maintenance. The most important coronary intervention is risk factor modification by *controlling blood pressure, lipid levels,* and *physical size and by stopping smoking.*

Primary prevention means preventing cardiovascular disease in the first place. Medical measures to prevent coronary heart disease in women are low-dose aspirin, taking cholesterol-lowering medicines, and, for those with elevated homocysteine levels, folate and Vitamins B12 and B6. Be careful not take more than 400 mcg of Vitamin E, as this has been correlated with increased clotting. In the Nurses' Health Study, aspirin 100 mg was associated with a 24 percent reduction in strokes caused by clots but only a 9 percent, nonsignificant, reduction in cardiovascular events (Ridker et al., 2005). I recommend aspirin 81 mg for my moderate and high-risk patients. Synthetic postmenopausal estrogens are not recommended for anyone to prevent heart disease since they appear to increase cardiovascular risk (Hulley et al., 1998; Roussow et al., 2002). High-risk postmenopausal women randomized as to hormone replacement had a 52 percent higher cardiac event rate in the first year of the study. Healthy postmenopasual women on hormone replacement had almost 30 percent higher cardiac event rates.

In my low-risk patients, I measure homocysteine once and fasting lipid profile every year. This interval shortens to three months for high-risk patients and to six weeks if I have modified therapy and want to check the results.

I encourage patients to try complete tobacco cessation, plus thirty minutes of aerobic exercise at least seven days a week if overweight and three times a week if normal weight. Walking is probably the best exercise, but this should not be a leisurely stroll. I used to tell patients to try to reach their maximal heart rate for their age, but now I tell them to try to quickly increase to a pace where it is difficult to carry on a conversation. Take the stairs and park the car in the farthest spot whenever possible. Try commuting to work by bicycle or public transportation. Try to get at least seven hours of sleep a night. Sleeping less than six hours a night is associated with decreased cognition, depressed mood, increased irritability, increased diabetes mellitus and obesity, increased infection, increased chronic fatigue syndrome, increased breast cancer incidence, and yes, increased coronary heart disease and hypertension. Remember, sleep is the most important time to rest and repair. Sleep deprivation creates hormonal imbalances such as increased cortisol or stress hormone levels, which may be the reason for the increase in cardiovascular disease (Ayas et al., 2003). Prayer and meditation have proven beneficial in managing the African American hypertensive patient (Walker et al., 2002).

Diet is a loaded subject in the African American community. The traditional high-fat, high-caloric African American diet was useful for a specific purpose—to provide energy to sustain a physically laborious lifestyle. One reason African American women have disproportionate obesity is trying to maintain a high-calorie diet while performing less exercise than their Caucasian counterparts. The American Heart Association therapeutic lifestyle change recommends most Americans reduce dietary fat intake to less than 30 percent total caloric intake, with 7 percent saturated fat, 10 percent polyunsaturated fat (vegetable oil), and 20 percent monounsaturated fat (olive oil), aiming for no more than 200 mg of cholesterol daily (American Heart Association, 2005). Remember to eat more of the good fats like olive oil and less of the bad or saturated fats like animal fats. Eat foods rich in omega 3 fatty acids and monounsaturated fats like olive oil (which is why that Mediterranean diet is so healthy), and avoid transfatty acids or partially hydrogenated oils like those found in many fast foods. If carnivorous, try to eat at least one meatless dinner a week and try to avoid meat at breakfast and lunch. Additional dietary measures include increasing plant sterol intake from things like tofu and other soybean preparations and increasing viscous soluble fiber like oatmeal. My diet plan consists of fruit sprinkled with raw oatmeal, a half slice of multigrain bread, and black coffee in the morning; apple and soup with salad or raw vegetables for lunch on most weekdays; and then a palm-sized portion of fish, chicken, pork, or beef in the evening, with two vegetables and a brown starch. Sometimes I snack on almonds or walnuts in the afternoon. I believe this satisfies the recently updated U.S. Department of Agriculture (USDA) recommendations of three to five servings of fruits and vegetables daily. I have personally used oatmeal, apples, and garlic to optimize my lipid profile without taking medications. A glass of red wine a night can raise HDL, but women should not drink more, particularly if taking certain medications, due to toxic effects on the liver. Other spirits have a similar effect, but a larger quantity is required. This means more calories and potential liver toxicity.

Do not forget to keep sodium intake low. Most of us should have no more than 2,400 mg daily, and less if we are already hypertensive. The Dietary Approaches to Stop Hypertension (DASH) diet can lower blood pressure by at least 5 mmHg (Douglas et al., 2003). It is important to read those labels.

All of these procedures and medicines have side effects but I tell my patients the risk is less than of a preventable death. Remember, the only way to prevent yourself from becoming a heart statistic is for you and your doctor to:

1. Keep blood pressure 120/80 and measure regularly, including at home and work.
2. Keep good cholesterol (HDL) greater than 40 (greater than 50 if you are a woman).
3. Keep bad cholesterol (LDL) less than 100 (70 if you have heart disease or diabetes).
4. Get tested for diabetes and keep your hemoglobin A1C at less than 6 percent.
5. Stop smoking and all other forms of tobacco.
6. Exercise seven days a week for at least twenty minutes if you are overweight, three times a week if not.
7. Get at least seven hours of sleep a night.
8. Drink at least six tall glasses of water a day.
9. Eat less and more selectively, with a complex carbohydrate (whole grain), low saturated fat, low-cholesterol, low-calorie diet—cut down on fast food intake; eat three to five fruits and three to five vegetables daily.
10. Keep your waist size less than 35 inches for woman and 40 inches for a man.
11. Follow your body mass index (normal: 20–25).
12. Know your C-reactive protein and homocysteine levels.
13. Discuss taking Vitamins B6 and B12, folate, aspirin, and alcohol with your doctor.
14. Do not think estrogens will prevent a heart attack, since they may do the opposite.
15. Know heart attack symptoms and ask for advanced testing if you have them.
16. When in the emergency room for heart problem, ask for an ECG and troponin-T.
17. If you have a heart attack, ask how the artery will be opened and when.
18. After the heart attack, ask for medicines to prevent another one.
19. After the heart attack, ask for cardiac rehabilitation and go there.
20. Do not stop the medicines suddenly.
21. Educate yourself about your disease and your doctor—know the guidelines and his or her board certification status.
22. Make sure your family also becomes educated.
23. Pray, meditate, or just appreciate quiet time.

REFERENCES

Ades, P. 2001. Cardiac Rehabilitation and Secondary Prevention of Coronary Heart Disease. *New England Journal of Medicine* 345(12):892–902.
American College of Cardiology. Guidelines for Management of ST Elevation MI. Available online at acc.org.

American Heart Association. *Heart Disease and Stroke Statistics—2005 Update.*
Ashen, et al. 2005. Low HDL Cholesterol Levels. *New England Journal of Medicine* 353:1252–60.
Ayas, et al. 2003. A Prospective Study of Sleep Duration and Coronary Heart Disease in Women. *Archives of Internal Medicine* 163:205–9.
Bild, D., et al. 2005. Ethnic Differences in Coronary Calcification. *Circulation* 111:1313–20.
Braunwald, E. 1997. Shattuck Lecture. *New England Journal of Medicine* 337:1360–69.
Budoff, M., et al. 2002. Ethnic Differences in Coronary Atherosclerosis. *Journal of the American College of Cardiology* 39:408–12.
Centers for Disease Control. 2004. *Morbidity and Mortality Weekly Review* 153:121–25.
Chobanian, Aram, George Bakris, Henry Black, et al. 2003. JNC VII Report. *Journal of the American Medical Association* 289:2560–72.
Collins, C. F. 2003. *Sources of Stress and Relief for African American Women*, pp. 8–9. Westport, Conn.: Praeger.
Crawford-Green, C. 1996. Hypertension and African American Women. In C. Collins, ed., *African American Women's Health and Social Issues*. Westport, Conn.: Praeger.
Douglas, J., et al. 2003. Management of High Blood Pressure in African Americans. *Archives of Internal Medicine* 163:525–41.
Gould, et al. 1998. *Circulation* 97:946–52.
Graham, et al. 2005. Risk of Acute Myocardial Infarction and Sudden Cardiac Death in Patients Treated with Cyclooxygenase 2 Selective and Nonselective Nonsteroidal Antiinflammatory Drugs. *Lancet* 365:475–81.
Grundy, et al. 2004. Implications of Recent Clinical Trials for the National Cholesterol Education Program Adult Treatment Panel 3 Guidelines. *Circulation* 110:227–39.
Healy, B. 1990. The Yentl Syndrome. *New England Journal of Medicine* 325(4):274–75.
Hochman, J., et al. 1999. Sex, Clinical Presentation and Outcome in Patients with Acute Coronary Syndromes. *New England Journal of Medicine* 341:226–32.
Hulley, et al. 1998. Randomized Trial of Estrogen plus Progestin for Secondary Prevention of Coronary Heart Disease in Women. *Journal of the American Medical Association* 280:605–13.
Jacobs, Bradley, Bernadette Boden, I-Feng Wn, et al. 2002. Stroke in the Young in the Northern Manhattan Stroke Study. *Stroke* 33:2789–93.
Jha, A., et al. 2005. Racial Trends in the Use of Major Procedures among the Elderly. *New England Journal of Medicine* 353(7):683–91.
Jha, Ashish, Elliott Fisher, Zhonghe Li, et al. 2003. Differences in Medical Care and Disease Outcomes among Black and White Women with Heart Disease. *Circulation* p. 108.
Johnston, S., et al. 2001. Utilization of Intravenous Tissue-Type Plasminogen Activator for Ischemic Stroke at Academic Medical Centers. *Stroke* 110(32):1061–68.
Keil, et al. 1993. Mortality Rates and Risk Factors for Coronary Disease in Black as Compared with White Men and Women. *New England Journal of Medicine* 329:73–78.
Lansky, A., et al. 2005. Percutaneous Coronary Intervention and Adjunctive Pharmacotherapy in Women. *Circulation* 111:940–53.
Lee, P., et al. 2001. Representation of Elderly Persons and Women in Published Randomized Trials of Acute Coronary Syndromes. *Journal of the American Medical Association* 286(6):708–13.
Levy, D., et al. 1990. Prognostic Implications of Echocardiographically Determined Left Ventricular Mass in the Framingham Heart Study. *New England Journal of Medicine* 322:1561–66.

Luft, Friedrich, et al. 1979. Cardiovascular and Humoral Responses to Extremes of Sodium Intake in Normal White and Black Men. *Circulation* 60:697.

Manson, JoAnn, Graham Colditz, Meir Stampfer, et al. 1990. Prospective Study of Obesity and Risk of Coronary Heart Disease in Women. *New England Journal of Medicine* 322:882–89.

Mensah, et al. 2005. State of Disparities in Cardiovascular Health in the United States. *Circulation* 111:1233–41.

Mieres, J., et al. 2005. Noninvasive Diagnosis of Coronary Heart Disease in Women. *Cardiology* (Special Section) 11:82–86.

Mosca, Lawrence Appel, Emelia Benjamin, Kathy Berra, et al. 2004a. Evidence-Based Guidelines for Cardiovascular Disease Prevention in Women. *Journal of the American College of Cardiology* 43:900–921.

Mosca, Lori, Anjanette Ferris, Rosalind Fabunmi, et al. 2004b. Tracking Women's Awareness of Heart Disease. *Circulation* 109:573–79.

Moses, et al. 2003. Sirolimus-Eluting Stents versus Standard Stents in Patients with Stenosis in a Native Coronary Artery. *New England Journal of Medicine* 349:1315–23.

National Cholesterol Education Program. Executive Summary of the Third Report of the National Cholesterol Education Program. *Journal of the American Medical Association* 285(19):2486–95.

National Institutes of Health. 1994. Guidelines on the Inclusion of Women and Minorities as Subjects in Clinical Research. *Federal Register* 59:11146.

Parmley, W. 2004. African American Patients and Heart Disease. *Circulation* 38(5):1577.

Petrie, K. 1999. Failure of Women's Hearts. *Circulation* 99:2334–41.

Pope, J., et al. 2000. Missed Diagnoses of Acute Cardiac Ischemia in the Emergency Department. *New England Journal of Medicine* 342:1163–70.

Racial/Ethnic Differences in Cardiac Care: The Weight of the Evidence. 2002. Henry J. Kaiser Family Foundation, American College of Cardiology Foundation, October.

Rich-Edwards, Janet, Joann Manson, Charles Hennekens, et al. 1995. Primary Prevention of Coronary Heart Disease in Women. *New England Journal of Medicine* 332(26):1758–63.

Ridker, Paul, Nancy Cook, I-Min Lee, et al. 2005. Randomized Trial of Low-Dose Aspirin in the Primary Prevention of Cardiovascular Disease in Women. *New England Journal of Medicine* 352:1293–304.

Ridker, Paul, Charles Hennekens, Julie Buring, et al. 2000. C-Reactive Protein and Other Markers of Inflammation in the Prediction of Cardiovascular Disease in Women. *New England Journal of Medicine* 342:836–43.

Rose, et al. 2001. Long-Term Use of a Left Ventricular Assist Device for End-Stage Heart Failure. *New England Journal of Medicine* 345:1435–43.

Ross, R. 1999. Atherosclerosis—An Inflammatory Disease. *New England Journal of Medicine* 340:115–26.

Roussow, et al. 2002. Risks and Benefits of Estrogen plus Progestin in Healthy Postmenopausal Women: Women's Health Initiative. *Journal of the American Medical Association* 288:321–33.

Saunders, Elijah. 1991. Cardiovascular Diseases in Blacks. *Cardiology Clinics of North America* 21(3):14.

Schneider, E., et al. 2001. Racial Differences in Cardiac Revascularization Rates. *Annals of Internal Medicine* 135:328–37.

Schnyder, G., et al. 2001. Decreased Rate of Coronary Restenosis after Lowering of Plasma Homocysteine Levels. *New England Journal of Medicine* 345(22):1593–600.

Schulman, K., et al. 1999. Effect of Race and Sex on Physicians' Recommendations for Cardiac Catheterization. *New England Journal of Medicine* 340:618–26.

Sonel, et al. 2005. Racial Variations in Treatment and Outcome of Black and White Patients with High-Risk Non-ST-Elevation Acute Coronary Syndromes. *Circulation* 111:1225–32.

Steffen, et al. 2003. Disparities in Premature Deaths from Heart Disease. *Psychosomatic Medicine* September/October.

Taylor, Anne, Susan Ziesche, Clyde Yancy, et al. 2004. Combination of Isosorbide Dinitrate and Hydralazine in Blacks with Heart Failure. *New England Journal of Medicine* 351:2049–57.

Walker, C., et al. 2002. Healing Power of Faith. *Journal of Urban Cardiology* 9(2):8–15.

Watson, K. 2005. Coronary Heart Disease in African Americans. *ABC Digest of Urban Cardiology* 31(1):33–35.

Wenger, et al. 1993. Cardiovascular Health and Disease in Women. *New England Journal of Medicine* 329:247–53.

Yancy, Clyde, Emeila Benjamin, Rosalind Fabunmi, et al. 2005. Discovering the Full Spectrum of Cardiovascular Disease. *Circulation* 111:1339–49.

Zacharias, et al. 2005. Operative and Late Coronary Artery Bypass Grafting Outcomes in Matched African-American versus Caucasian Patients. *Journal of the American College of Cardiology* 46(8):1526–35.

2

Breast Cancer in African American Women

PATRICIA K. BRADLEY

Breast cancer is a disease of abnormal growth and spread of cells in the form of a tumor in the breast. Although breast cancer can occur in men, it most commonly occurs in women. Much remains unknown about the disease of breast cancer, including where it comes from and how to prevent it. What *is* known about breast cancer does not portray an encouraging picture as it relates to African American women. Breast cancer is the second leading cause of cancer death among African American women. African American women are at high risk for both a greater mortality rate and a presentation for cancer treatment at a later stage of disease. Although the incidence rate of breast cancer is about 17 percent lower in African American women than in white women, the death rate is 32 percent higher (American Cancer Society [ACS], 2005). This difference in death rates remains, even with increased efforts to improve survival through the development of effective detection techniques and an increase in the number of possible treatment options (Bradley et al., 2001).

The five-year relative survival rate for breast cancer diagnosed from 1995 to 2000 among African American women was 75 percent, compared with 89 percent among whites (ACS, 2005). In fact, African American women with breast cancer continue to be more likely to die often than any other group of women (Li et al., 2003). A number of causes have been considered for the survival differences between African American and white American women. Disproportionate breast cancer deaths in African American women have been linked to: (1) low socioeconomic status; (2) specific biological characteristics of the tumor such as tumor grade and estrogen receptivity; (3) younger age at diagnosis (younger than 45); (4) multiple coexisting medical conditions, particularly for older women; (5) delay in diagnosis and treatment; (6) treatment differences; and (7) differences in access to early detection and prompt treatment

(Chu et al., 2003; Joslyn & West, 2000; Long, 1993). Any of these factors can lead to an advanced stage of the disease at diagnosis. Advanced stage is indicated by increased tumor size, tumor stage at diagnosis, and an increased number of positive axillary lymph nodes (Moormeier, 1996; Rose & Royak-Schaler, 2001). The one factor most often associated with African American women's advanced stage is delay in seeking treatment (Facione, 1993; Lannin et al., 1998; Phillips & Smith, 2001).

SEEKING TREATMENT FOR BREAST CANCER

Delay in seeking treatment for breast cancer symptoms is mostly viewed as being patient initiated. African Americans' fatalistic attitudes and distrust of the health care system are the two patient-related characteristics most often linked to delay in seeking treatment (Conrad et al., 1996; Powe & Finnie, 2003). Emotional barriers to getting care that may lead to delay include a lack of knowledge about breast cancer, an inaccurate perception of the risk of breast cancer, and the belief that breast cancer screening examinations are necessary only if a lump is detected (Gates et al., 2001).

The fact is that screening for breast cancer before symptoms appear increases the chance that the cancer will be detected early. Detection of breast cancer at an early stage provides diagnosed women with the greatest probability of survival. The detection of breast cancer consists of medical interventions including mammography screening and diagnosis, monitoring, and follow-up of ambiguous or suspicious findings with breast biopsy. The American Cancer Society (2005) recommends that women over 40 get an annual mammogram and an annual clinical breast examination (CBE) of the breast by a health care provider. Women are also encouraged to be familiar with the appearance and feel of their breasts to note for any changes that may need follow-up by a health professional. Particular patient-related barriers to screening that have been identified are the perception of mammograms as painful and uncomfortable and the fear of negative (cancer diagnosis) or unreliable results (Adams et al., 2001; Williams et al., 1997).

Individual, patient-initiated barriers are not the sole contributors to delay in seeking treatment. Health care system barriers that may lead to African American women delaying include differences in access to preventive health care and to early detection and prompt treatment; inadequate continuity of care; the inconvenience of health care facilities' available hours, days, and location; the cost of the service; and a lack of transportation (Caplan et al., 1996; Williams et al., 1997). However, these factors are not often examined as contributing to delay (Farmer & Smith, 2002; Smith et al., 2001) as the major focus of research, and programmatic interventions continue to be on individual actions.

In a study of African American women's psychosocial responses to breast cancer symptoms, P. K. Bradley (2005) found that the women who were least likely to delay seeking diagnosis and treatment for breast cancer symptoms had particular characteristics that matched those of white women who do not delay (Coates et al., 1992). Those who did not delay reported having a regular source of medical care providing them access to treatment and a relationship with a health provider. Participants also reported having a source of support from participation in organizations such as attendance at church, and knowledge about cancer and detection procedures. Similarly, Mitchell et al. (2002) found that women who reported timely breast cancer screenings were more likely to have full health insurance coverage, knowledge about breast cancer risk factors, and involvement in the health care system. Additionally, contrary to other studies reporting fatalistic beliefs of African Americans about cancer (Conrad et al., 1996; Jennings, 1996; Phillips et al., 1999; Powe & Finnie, 2003), the majority of participants believed that their symptom was something that could be taken care of (Bradley, 2005).

The significance of these findings is that when African American women are given adequate information and appropriate resources, they are more likely to identify breast cancer symptoms and to get prompt treatment for them. Increased participation in routine mammography screening, with subsequent detection and treatment of the disease at an early stage, offers the best opportunity for decreasing mortality and improving survival. To benefit from early detection, African American women must have access to these methods.

Racism as a Barrier

Racism is a significant system-related barrier resulting in delayed seeking of treatment. For African Americans, perceived or actual differences in treatment contribute to the perception of racism in the health care system. Perceived racism as defined by Green (1995) is the individual's judgment that racism exists. She posits that an individual perceives differential treatment, experiences, or attitudes and acts on the basis of these perceptions. Essed (1991) and Feagin and Sikes (1994) described experiences of racism for African Americans as cumulative, with new encounters interpreted on the basis of past experiences with racism, knowledge of other's experiences with racism, such as the Tuskegee Syphilis Study (Gamble, 1993), and knowledge about the systemic nature of racism. Green (1995) suggests that this racism is perceived on affective (feelings), behavioral (actions), and cognitive (thoughts) levels. The challenge for researchers, clinicians, and educators is to understand the historically based realities and the impact of events for the individual that underlie African Americans' sentiments of distrust of the health care system, providers, and research.

Racism is an exemplar of the historical and cultural experiences of African American women that may negatively influence participation in cancer-related activities and may also result in African Americans delaying seeking health care. In addition to the injustice of the frequently cited Tuskegee Study, findings from other research with African American people have demonstrated the spheres of racism.

Osborne and Feit (1992) described the racism inherent in the use of race as a variable in medical research and the implied assumption that a genetic reason may explain differences in incidence, severity, or outcome of medical conditions. The implication and subtle racism here is the assumed genetic superiority of the racial group with the least incidence of the disease or better outcome.

Results of Black/white comparison research in which differences in outcomes are noted for African Americans are often interpreted as negative. Whites are often held as the standard of normalcy and universality, while Blacks are viewed as pathological to the extent that they deviate from the norm (Barbee, 1994).

Labeling African Americans as inferior or pathological because they differ from white Americans is a form of subtle racism often exhibited in research. Efforts to include more African Americans in clinical trials and to develop community-collaborative research programs must address the legacy of distrust brought about by the exploitive actions of medical researchers. This distrust is sometimes dismissed as paranoia or hypersensitivity. However, Grier and Cobbs (1968) referred to these emotions as "healthy cultural paranoia" based on the real experiences of racism and discrimination.

In the past, access to research studies has been limited for African Americans and other socioeconomically disadvantaged groups because the trials were selective due to their design, geographical location, type of institution used, and a lack of awareness of the importance of broad representation (Outlaw et al., 2000). The generalizability of clinical trial results depends on how restricted the study sample has been and the nature of the restrictions. The effect of the Tuskegee Study of creating a distrustful relationship between the African American community and the scientific community has created a paradox for African Americans. That is, African Americans are disproportionately represented in mortality and morbidity statistics for medical problems such as cancer; they are, however, underrepresented in treatment and prevention trials. Therefore, data are less generalizable to African Americans, making the effectiveness of new interventions in this population unknown. African American women who have stated their interests in participation in clinical studies have reported that a significant barrier to participation has been their not being asked to participate by their providers (Freedman, 1998; Millon-Underwood et al., 1993).

Acknowledging African American women's experience with racism and understanding the influence racism has on perceptions of health and illness is a crucial step for health providers in developing trustworthy relationships and providing culturally appropriate interventions (Outlaw, 1993). In the case of breast cancer and African Americans, perceived racism may play a factor in underutilization of screening activities, influencing African American women's delayed seeking of care and subsequent negative health outcomes.

Addressing Barriers

Accessible services are services that are physically available, economically attainable, culturally acceptable, qualitatively appropriate, and nondiscriminatory (Campinha-Bacote, 1994). Access, whether perceived or actual, is an important part of seeking care. Receiving adequate health care is dependent on having a health provider. One does not always guarantee the other, however, nor does having medical coverage ensure access to quality medical care (Shavers & Brown, 2002).

In 2003, the National Academy of Sciences' Institute of Medicine (IOM) released a report that underscores this point (Smedley et al., 2003). The IOM is a private, nonprofit institution that provides health policy advice under a congressional charter granted to the National Academy of Science. This comprehensive report of the IOM, which reviewed over a hundred studies conducted over the last ten years, found that racial and ethnic minorities in the United States receive lower quality health care than whites, even when their insurance, income, age, and severity of condition are similar. The major recommendation for reducing racial and ethnic disparities in health care was to increase awareness among the general public, health care providers, insurance companies, and policymakers regarding these disparities. The IOM report (Smedley et al., 2003) also calls for the promotion of consistency and equity of care through the use of "evidence-based" guidelines. These guidelines would help providers and health insurers make decisions about which procedures to order or pay for based on the best available science.

Currently interventions with African American women are primarily designed to address individual behavioral barriers to care. To remain at this level of intervention without addressing social policy and provider issues puts the sole responsibility for change on the individual. Individual, provider, and social policy levels of intervention must be addressed to impact the health delivery system and to increase access for African Americans. We must identify the barriers to access and must advocate change on the health policy and health provider levels, directed toward assuring access to quality care for all individuals (Phillips & Smith, 2001).

Health care providers play an important role in connecting African American women to screening, treatment, support, and breast cancer education. Negative health encounters are significant practitioner-related barriers to African American women seeking prompt treatment and follow-up care (Ashing-Giwa & Ganz, 1997; Barg & Gullatte, 2001). Behavioral interventions directed toward health providers and African American women must include education to increase knowledge of the efficacy and availability of early detection activities as well as addressing personal emotions. Health care providers' culturally sensitive and trustworthy interactions are needed to help in addressing the barriers of discrimination and racism present in the existing system. Getting all health care providers to recommend mammography, to perform clinical breast exams, and to encourage women to be familiar with their breasts and any changes, is essential to increasing African American women's screening behaviors. Addressing the barriers to inclusion of African American women into both prevention and treatment clinical trials is imperative to allow for findings regarding the effectiveness of new interventions to be generalized to this population (Jones & Chilton, 2002; Underwood, 2003).

COPING WITH A BREAST CANCER DIAGNOSIS

Until recently, little has been written about the coping skills of African American women in response to a breast cancer diagnosis. African Americans have been using spirituality and religion for generations as effective resources for coping with both illness and adversity (Gibson, 2003; Newlin et al., 2002; Outlaw, 1993). Studies examining explanatory models for health beliefs in general, and cancer specifically, among African Americans have uncovered salient themes of spirituality as a way of coping with illness (Gregg & Curry, 1994; Mitchel et al., 2001; Potts, 1996; Moore, 2001; Reynolds et al., 2000; Roberson, 1985).

Most African Americans seek help from extended family members, very close family friends, ministers, and church leaders (Bailey, 1987; Billingsley, 1992). Quite often, only after exhausting available inner, familial, and spiritual resources does the person seek medical advice. This cultural model of care seeking, as identified by Bailey (1987), has been characterized as a form of delay (Hoffman-Goetz & Mills, 1997), however it is also a self-care model that can be considered when planning intervention projects. Religion can and has been used as a support component to change health behaviors of African Americans. Boyd-Franklin (1989) views the church as a more concrete manifestation of the widespread spiritual orientation in African American families, as many African Americans have used the Black church community experience as a major coping mechanism in handling the overwhelming pain of racism and discrimination.

Gregg and Curry (1994) and others (Ashing-Giwa & Ganz, 1997; Northouse et al., 1999) also found that for a number of women, their faith in God and their health behavior were inextricably connected; God was cited as a reason to see the doctors as well as the reason the doctors succeeded with treatments. Holt et al. (2003) described this spiritual health locus of control (SHLOC) as having two dimensions: active and passive. Active SHLOC empowers individuals, through their health beliefs and behaviors, to take an active role in determining their health outcomes. Passive SHLOC, on the other hand, involves reliance on a higher power such as God to protect their health. Understanding the significance of African Americans' strong faith in God and His Will to provide the necessary means, such as trained physicians and treatments, as well as the central place the church has in establishing and supporting these beliefs, is essential to effectively reaching and working with African American women.

Not all African American women perceive breast cancer as an automatic death sentence. In a project to develop educational materials for African American women (Bradley et al., 1999), focus groups were used to explore African American women's thoughts and concerns about surviving and living beyond a breast cancer diagnosis. African American women expressed the belief that effective coping is possible through connection to five areas: self, God or nature, family and friends, other survivors, and the health care treatment team. The process used to make this connection involves surviving the impact of hearing the diagnosis, making decisions about treatment, relating to others for support, and living beyond breast cancer through follow-up with health providers. African American breast cancer survivors expressed the belief that living after a breast cancer diagnosis is possible through the use of spirituality, informed decision making, developing and maintaining positive connections, and reaching out to others for support and with encouragement. This is quite similar to the findings of Henderson et al. (2003) and Northouse et al. (1999), in which African American women reported a high quality of life and positive family functioning following diagnosis. Major factors enabling this coping were the positive connections, expression of emotions, and the use of spirituality.

African American women have defined having a culturally congruent support network to assist with emotions evoked by a breast cancer diagnosis as including spiritual expression (Barg & Gullatte, 2001; Henderson & Fogel, 2003). The portrayal of positive coping in the media and use of culturally sensitive approaches have also been identified as key strategies to connect women to care and to decrease cancer fatalism (Moore, 2001; Northouse et al., 1999; Williams-Brown et al., 2002). Additionally, African American women surviving breast cancer are often motivated through their experiences with breast cancer to reach out to others, in what Wilmoth and Sanders (2001) have termed "health activism." Participants in their study sought to help other women to be more aware of their risk and of breast cancer screening methods.

SUMMARY

There are many unknowns about breast cancer. What is known is that finding the cancer at an early stage and doing something about it right away offers the best chance of a positive outcome for women diagnosed with breast cancer. What is also known about breast cancer is that women who have supportive services, including access and referrals to screenings, adequate treatment resources, and positive relationships with health care providers, are more likely to seek care promptly than those without.

To increase the survival rate of African American women diagnosed with breast cancer, it is imperative that health professionals become more involved in assuring access to early detection methods. It is important to explore our setting for structures that foster prejudice and discrimination, identifying and eliminating access and availability of services barriers and advocating policy changes. Increasing the number of positive health care encounters and the sensitivity and cultural appropriateness in treatment environments may increase the likelihood of African American women seeking treatment earlier, the probability of survival, and the improvement of the quality of care. Survivors can be assisted in positive coping through supportive networks that include connectedness and an openness to spirituality. Research and program development tailored to African American women must also take into consideration additional burdens and institutional and health policy barriers.

REFERENCES

Adams, M. L., H. Becker, and A. Colbert. 2001. African-American women's perceptions of mammography screening. *Journal of the National Black Nurses Association,* 12, 44–48.

American Cancer Society. 2005. *Cancer Facts and Figures for African Americans 2005–2006.* Atlanta, GA: Author.

Ashing-Giwa, K., and P. Ganz. 1997. Understanding the breast cancer experience of African American women. *Journal of Psychosocial Oncology,* 15, 19–35.

Bailey, E. J. 1987. Sociocultural factors and health care-seeking behavior among Black Americans. *Journal of the American Medical Association*, 79, 3899–3902.

Barbee, E. L. 1994. A black feminist approach to nursing research. *Western Journal of Nursing Research*, 16, 495–506.

Barg, F., and M. Gullatte. 2001. Cancer support groups: Meeting the needs of African Americans with cancer. *Seminars in Oncology Nursing*, 17, 171–178.

Billingsley, A. 1992. *Climbing Jacob's ladder: The enduring legacy of African American families*. New York: Simon & Schuster.

Boyd-Franklin, N. 1989. *Black Families in Therapy: A Multisystems Approach*. New York: Guilford.

Bradley, C. J., C. W. Given, and C. Roberts. 2001. Disparities in cancer diagnosis. *Journal of the American Medical Association*, 287, 2106–2113.

Bradley, P. K. 2005. The delay and worry experience of African American women with breast cancer. *Oncology Nursing Forum*, 32, 243–249.

Bradley P. K., and M. N. Scharf. 1999. Living beyond breast cancer. *Getting Connected: African Americans Living beyond Breast Cancer*. Ardmore Pa.: Living Beyond Breast Cancer.

Campinha-Bacote, J. 1994. *The Process of Cultural Competence in Health Care: A Culturally Competent Model of Care*. Wyoming, OH: Perfect Printing Press.

Caplan, L. S., K. J. Helzlsouer, S. Shapiro, M. N. Wesley, and B. K. Edwards. 1996. Reasons for delay in breast cancer diagnosis. *Preventive Medicine*, 25, 218–224.

Chu, K. C., C. A. Lamar, and H. P. Freeman. 2003. Racial disparities in breast carcinoma survival rates: Separating factors that affect diagnosis from factors that affect treatment. *Cancer*, 97, 2853–2860.

Coates, R. J., D. D. Bransfields, M. N. Wesley, B. Hankey, J. W. Eley, R. S. Greenberg, et al. 1992. Differences between black and white women with breast cancer in time from symptom recognition to medical consultation. *Journal of the National Cancer Institute*, 84, 938–950.

Conrad, M. E., P. Brown, and M. G. Conrad. 1996. Fatalism and breast cancer in black women. *Annals of Internal Medicine*, 125, 941–942.

Essed, P. 1991. *Understanding Everyday Racism: An Interdisciplinary Theory*. Newbury Park, CA: Sage Publications.

Facione, N. C. 1993. Delay versus helpseeking for breast cancer symptoms: A critical review of the literature on patient and provider delay. *Social Science and Medicine*, 36, 1521–1534.

Farmer, B. J., and E. D. Smith. 2002. Breast cancer survivorship: Are African American women considered? A concept analysis. *Oncology Nursing Forum*, 29, 770–787.

Feagin, J. R., and M. P. Sikes. 1994. *Living with Racism: The Black Middle-Class Experience*. Boston: Beacon Press.

Freedman, T. 1998. Why don't they come to Pike Street and ask us? Black women's health concerns. *Social Science and Medicine*, 47, 941–947.

Gamble, V. N. 1993. A legacy of distrust: African Americans and medical research. *American Journal of Preventive Medicine*, 9, 35–38.

Gates, M. F., N. R. Lackey, and G. Brown. 2001. Caring demands and delay in seeking care in African American women newly diagnosed with breast cancer: An ethnographic, photographic study. *Oncology Nursing Forum*, 28, 529–537.

Gibson L. M. 2003. Inter-relationships among sense of coherence, hope, and spiritual perspective (inner resources) of African American breast cancer survivors. *Applied Nursing Research*, 16, 236–244.

Green, N. 1995. Development of the perceptions of racism scale. *Image: Journal of Nursing Scholarship,* 27, 141–146.

Gregg, J., and R. H. Curry. 1994. Explanatory models for cancer among African American women at two Atlanta neighborhood health centers: The implications for a cancer screening program. *Social Science and Medicine,* 39, 519–526.

Grier, W., and P. Cobbs. 1968. *Black Rage.* New York: Basic Books.

Henderson, P. D., and J. Fogel. 2003. Support networks used by African American breast cancer support group participants. *The Association of Black Nursing Faculty Journal,* 15, 95–98.

Henderson, P. D., J. Fogel, and Q. Edwards. 2003. Coping strategies among African American women with breast cancer. *Southern Online Journal of Nursing Research,* 3, 1–20.

Henderson, P. D., S. V. Gore, B. L. Davis, and E. Condon. 2003. African American women coping with breast cancer: A qualitative analysis. *Oncology Nursing Forum,* 30, 641–646.

Hoffman-Goetz, L., and S. L. Mills. 1997. Cultural barriers to cancer screening among African American women: A critical review of the qualitative literature. *Women's Health: Research on Gender, Behavior, and Policy,* 3, 183–201.

Holt, C. L., E. M. Clark, M. W. Kreuter, and D. M. Rubio. 2003. Spiritual health locus of control and breast cancer beliefs among urban African American women. *Health Psychology,* 22, 294–299.

Jennings, K. 1996. Getting black women to screen for cancer: Incorporating health beliefs into practice. *Journal of the American Academy of Nurse Practitioners,* 8, 53–59.

Jones, L. A., and J. A. Chilton. 2002. Impact of breast cancer on African American women: Priority areas for research in the next decade. *American Journal of Public Health,* 92, 539–542.

Joslyn, S., and M. West. 2000. Racial differences in breast carcinoma survival. *Cancer,* 88, 114–123.

Lackey, N. R., M. F. Gates, and G. Brown. 2001. African American women's experiences with the initial discovery, diagnosis, and treatment of breast cancer. *Oncology Nursing Forum,* 28, 519–527.

Lannin, D. R., H. F. Mathews, J. Mitchell, M. S. Swanson, F. H. Swanson, and M. S. Edwards. 1998. Influence of socioeconomic and cultural factors on racial differences in late-stage presentation of breast cancer. *Journal of the American Medical Association,* 279, 1801–1807.

Li, C. I., K. M. Malone, and J. R. Daling. 2003. Differences in breast cancer stage, treatment, and survival by race and ethnicity. *Archives of Internal Medicine,* 163, 49–56.

Long, E. 1993. Breast cancer in African-American women: Review of the literature. *Cancer Nursing,* 16, 1–24.

Mathews, H. F., D. R. Lannin, and J. P. Mitchell. 1994. Coming to terms with advanced breast cancer: Black women's narratives from Eastern North Carolina. *Social Science and Medicine,* 38, 789–800.

Millon-Underwood, S., E. Sanders, and M. Davis. 1993. Determinants of participation in state-of-the art cancer prevention, early detection/screening, and treatment trials among African Americans. *Cancer Nursing,* 16, 25–33.

Mitchell, J., D. D. Lannin, H. F. Mathews, and M. S. Swanson. 2002. Religious beliefs and breast cancer screening. *Journal of Women's Health,* 11, 907–915.

Moore, R. J. 2001. African American women and breast cancer: Notes from a study narrative. *Cancer Nursing,* 24, 35–42.

Moormeier, J. 1996. Breast cancer in black women. *Annals of Internal Medicine,* 124, 897–905.

Newlin, K., K. Knafl, and G. Melkus. 2002. African-American spirituality: Concept analysis. *Advances in Nursing Science,* 25, 57–70.

Northouse, L. L., M. Caffey, L. Deichelbohrer, L. Schmidt, L. Guziatek-Trojniak, S. West, T. Kershaw, and D. Mood. 1999. The quality of life of African American women with breast cancer. *Research in Nursing and Health,* 22, 449–460.

Osborne, N. G., and M. D. Feit. 1992. The use of race in medical research. *Jama,* 267, 275–279.

Outlaw, F. H. 1993. Stress and coping: The influence of racism on the cognitive appraisal processing of African American. *Issues in Mental Health Nursing,* 14, 399–409.

Outlaw, F. H., J. N. Bourjolly, and F. K. Barg. 2000. A study of recruitment of Black Americans into clinical trials through a cultural competence lens. *Cancer Nursing,* 23, 444–451.

Phillips, J., and E. D. Smith. 2001. Breast cancer control and African American women: A review. *Cancer Investigation,* 19, 273–280.

Phillips, J. M., M. Z. Cohen, and G. Moses. 1999. Breast cancer screening and African American women: Fear, fatalism, and silence. *Oncology Nursing Forum,* 26, 561–571.

Potts, R. G. 1996. Spirituality and the experience of cancer in an African American community: Implications for psychosocial oncology. *Journal of Psychosocial Oncology,* 14(1):1–19.

Powe, B. D., and R. Finnie. 2003. Cancer fatalism: The state of the science. *Cancer Nursing,* 26, 454–465.

Reynolds, P., S. Hurley, M. Torres, J. Jackson, P. Boyd, V. W. Chen, et al. 2000. Use of coping strategies and breast cancer survival: Results from the black/white cancer survival study. *American Journal of Epidemiology,* 152, 940–949.

Roberson, M.H.B. 1985. The influence of religious beliefs on health choices of Afro-Americans. *Topics in Clinical Nursing,* 7(3):57–63.

Rose, D. P., and R. Royak-Schaler. 2001. Tumor biology and prognosis in black breast cancer patients: A review. *Cancer Detection and Prevention,* 25, 16–31.

Shavers, V. L., and M. L. Brown. 2002. Racial and ethnic disparities in the receipt of cancer treatment. *Journal of the National Cancer Institute,* 94, 334–357.

Smedley, B. D., A. Y. Stith, and A. R. Nelson. (Eds.) 2003. *Unequal treatment: Confronting racial and ethnic disparities in health care.* Washington, DC: National Academies Press.

Smith, E. D., J. M. Phillips, and M. H. Price. 2001. Breast cancer screening and early detection among racial and ethnic minority women. *Seminars in Oncology Nursing,* 17, 159–170.

Underwood, S. M. 2003. Reducing the burden of cancer borne by African American: If not now, when? *Cancer Epidemiology, Biomarkers and Prevention,* 12, 270–276.

Williams, G. A., R. R. Abbott, and D. K. Taylor. 1997. Using focus group methodology to develop breast cancer screening programs that recruit African American women. *Journal of Community Health,* 22(1):45–56.

Williams-Brown, S., S.D.M. Baldwin, and A. Bakos. 2002. Storytelling as a method to teach African American women breast health information. *Journal of Cancer Education,* 17, 227–230.

Wilmoth, M. C., and D. S. Sanders. 2001. Accept me for myself: African American women's issues after breast. *Oncology Nursing Forum,* 28, 875–879.

3

Understanding Sickle Cell Disease in African American Women

JAMESETTA A. NEWLAND
AND CASSANDRA DOBSON

Many African Americans have heard the term "bad blood." The stigma associated with these words has plagued African Americans since the times of slavery, before the term was created. Over the years individuals thought to have "bad blood" have been described with such adjectives as *weak, syphilitic, tainted*, and *unclean*; but most strikingly "of the Negro or black race." The phrase has been used as a weapon to label and discriminate against a race of people, based on the color of their skin or their assumed ancestry. Such treatment has created a health care system of inequality and disparities in access to care and ultimately in health status for the African American population compared to the white population.

In ignorance, "bad blood" has been used interchangeably with *sickle cell disease* (SCD), in the past called *sickle cell anemia*, a term for a group of genetic disorders characterized by the production of abnormal hemoglobin S, anemia, and acute and chronic tissue damage. After Congress passed the National Sickle Cell Anemia Control Act (1972), African Americans continued to receive misinformation about SCD during national campaigns to educate the Black community and encourage testing for the disease. There was much misunderstanding about the implications of the sickle cell trait, which is not classified as a type of SCD but has significant reproductive implications for African Americans.

Complications of SCD vary from individual to individual and encompass the full life span, often beginning within months of the birth of an affected infant. It is a disease characterized by chronicity and uncertainty, with periods of relative wellness interrupted by periods of serious illness and crises, frequently without warning and too often fatal. Individuals with SCD, however, no longer die in childhood or adolescence but rather live well into adulthood. African American women with SCD and sickle cell trait must make difficult decisions concerning reproduction: contraception, conception, genetic counseling and testing, and whether to abort or carry to term an affected fetus. Many women do not receive adequate information about SCD and are therefore not equipped with the necessary knowledge to manage SCD that affects themselves or a family member.

PURPOSE

In this chapter, the physical and psychosocial aspects of SCD on those affected is discussed, including the impact of the disease on the African American woman across the life span, with an emphasis on reproductive concerns and issues during pregnancy. Often it is the mother in a family who bears the greatest responsibility of meeting the needs of a child with SCD and of preparing that child to one day manage the disease. Therefore, it is important for African American women to understand all aspects of SCD. A historical recounting of the discovery of SCD and, separately, the influences of racism, stigmatism, and discrimination against African Americans in general is reported. A brief overview of the science is provided to add to understanding the integral relationship of the pathophysiology of SCD to manifestations and complications of the disease and to understand its transmission from one generation to the next. Psychosocial implications of SCD and strategies for coping with personal and family stress are introduced, of which self-advocacy is an important element. Therapeutic options for the treatment of SCD, both medical and nonmedical, are outlined. African American women owe it to themselves, their daughters, and female relatives and friends to learn as much as possible about SCD. Increased awareness about SCD and knowledge of the disease will benefit all African American women and their families, helping them make responsible decisions and lead healthy lives.

BACKGROUND

History of the Discovery of SCD in the United States

Dr. James Herrick published the first formal report of "peculiar elongated and sickle-shaped" cells in 1910, establishing the *clinical diagnosis* of sickled cells (Herrick, 1910). He and a hospital intern, Dr. Ernest Irons, discovered the abnormally shaped red cells in the blood of a twenty-year-old black dental student from the West Indies. Dr. Herrick had been attending him during multiple hospital admissions for illnesses over a two-and-a-half-year period, most frequently for severe anemia and repeated episodes of swollen joints and pain. More than sixty years prior to that, however, landowners had noticed that certain slaves were sickly and had less stamina than others. One report details physicians' perplexity at the absence of a spleen during the autopsy of a murdered runaway slave (Lebby, 1846). *Laboratory diagnosis* was introduced in 1917 through a crude test that demonstrated changes in the blood (sickling) when it was covered and deprived of air (oxygen). This highly inaccurate test was to become the standard for diagnosis during the next several decades. Belief that transmission from one generation to the next occurred through one parent also prevailed for more than thirty years. During this time, the term *sickle cell anemia* (SCA) was coined, associations between clinical symptoms and physical findings became more evident, and the distinction between disease (SCA) and nondisease (sickle cell trait) was clarified (Bullock & Jilly, 1975; Feldman & Tauber, 1997; Lessin & Jensen, 1974; Wailoo, 1991, 1997).

The development of electrophoretic techniques in the laboratory led the way for the discovery of *molecular disease*, SCD being the first (Pauling et al., 1949). The *genetic mutation* responsible for SCD was discovered in 1957, and the actual gene was isolated in 1977 (Wailoo, 1997). Science had finally proven false past theories of "bad blood" in the Negro race. Despite these discoveries, SCD did not receive the national attention it warranted.

Social Issues

Health disparities have always existed within and across groups of Americans, but are most visible when the health of racial and ethnic minorities is considered. African Americans are disproportionately more disadvantaged than whites (Williams-Morris, 1996). After the National Sickle Cell Anemia Control Act of 1972 was enacted, mass screening programs were organized by the government. Unfortunately, the response was less than desired. Screening programs were confusing to the public because objectives were not clearly stated and understood; there was confusion between trait and disease status, and educational and counseling programs were not always in place to interpret test results. Mistrust pervaded the Black community. Accusations were made by various public groups that the programs involved Black genocide. The Tuskegee experiment was fresh in the minds of Blacks (Chestnut, 1994). A few examples of the psychosocial effects of the early SCD programs experienced by Blacks were: (1) anxiety, fear, and apprehension because of inaccurate diagnosis by physicians and inaccurate and unduly alarming communication materials; (2) threat of destruction of families due to the potential for uncovering paternity; (3) anger and resentment as a result of increased insurance premiums, rejection for employment, and testing without consent; and (4) inhibition to the development of racial pride because of the perpetuation of a white paternalistic approach and inadequate funding to the Black community (Whitten & Fischhoff, 1974).

Today, with the successful mapping of the human genome and the ensuing implications of the genetic revolution, doubts exist about the equitable access to and distribution of genetic services to minority and disadvantaged groups in the United States. This new information is potentially lifesaving, while at the same time very threatening to groups without knowledge and power. Public education and advocacy will hopefully balance the scales. African American women can start by gaining an understanding of SCD, a disease that in the United States affects primarily people of African descent.

Statistics of Prevalence and Incidence

The gene is the basic unit of heredity. An allele is one of the possible alternative forms of a gene. Multiple alleles may exist for one gene but individuals carry only two alleles of a particular gene. Genotype refers to the specific allelic makeup of an individual for some characteristic.

Hemoglobin (two alpha and two beta chains) is the predominant protein in red blood cells. Mutations in structure or production in these chains results in hematological disease. The inheritance of two abnormal hemoglobin alleles in the beta chain results in sickle cell disease (SCD). The four most common genotypes in the United States are:

SCD-SS, two hemoglobin S genes or homozygous (the same alleles)

SCD-SC, one each of hemoglobin S and C

SCD-Sβ^+, one hemoglobin S and decreased production in beta chains

SCD-Sβ^0, one hemoglobin S and no production in beta chains

Although SCD affects primarily African Americans in the United States, worldwide, individuals of Mediterranean, Caribbean, South and Central American, Chinese, Middle Eastern, and East Indian ethnicity are affected. The incidence in Caucasians is very low. Exact statistics vary, depending on the source (Platt & Sacerdote, 2002), but these are numbers commonly cited for the United States:

- 1 in every 375 live African American (AA) births has homozygous SCD-SS.
- 1 in every 835 AA live births has SCD-SC.
- 1 in every 1,667 AA live births has sickle β-thalassemia.
- SCD affects between 50,000 and 70,000 AA.
- 1 in every 58,000 Caucasians in the U.S. population has some form of SCD.

Sickle cell trait occurs more frequently and affects more people:

- It occurs in 8 percent of all people of African descent.
- Sickle cell trait is found in people of Mediterranean descent.
- Sickle cell trait was transported to Europe from the Caribbean.
- In some areas equatorial Africa, as much as 60 percent of the population has sickle cell trait.

Morbidity and Mortality

As recent as the 1960s, SCD was considered a "disease of childhood." By 1973, the average life span of an individual with SCD-SS was approximately 14 years. Survival increased to 20 years for individuals with sickle thalassemias (100 percent); at 20 years survival is 85 percent in those with SCD-SS and 95 percent in those with SCD-SC. By 1994 (Platt et al., 1994), the median age of death for individuals with SCD-SS was 42 years and 48 years for males and females, respectively, and 60 years and 68 years for males and females with SCD-SC. Affected individuals now live well into adulthood. As they transition to independence and adult care, adolescents with SCD need the same guidance and instruction as unaffected adolescents.

Definition

SCD is a term for a group of genetic disorders characterized by production of hemoglobin S, anemia, and acute and chronic tissue damage secondary to the blockage of blood flow produced by abnormally shaped red cells. The disease is classified in the general category of hemoglobinopathies or conditions of abnormal hemoglobin.

Etiology

Sickle cell disease is the most common hemoglobin disorder in individuals of African descent worldwide. Although there are several theories to explain the origin of the sickle cell gene, a widely accepted one relates the presence of malaria in Africa as a plausible influence on the development of the sickle cell mutation. Selective resistance to malaria in individuals with sickle cell trait made them more likely to survive, have children, and pass on the gene. Individuals with SCD infected by the *Anopheles* mosquito, however, were more likely to die from complications of malaria, secondary to dehydration, fever, vaso-occlusion (blockage in blood vessels), and hyperhemolysis, or increased rupturing of red blood cells. The sickle cell mutation facilitated the seemingly uncontrollable replication and survival of the gene (Edelstein, 1986).

Genetics

Genes are the basic units of inheritance. They are located on chromosomes, which are structures in cells that contain the complex DNA codes (string of proteins), which are the chemical bases of heredity. Each person has 46 chromosomes in their cells, 26 donated from each parent. SCD is the result of a structural abnormality in the blood with a gene mutation on chromosome 11. Red blood cells (RBCs) contain the hemoglobin molecule, which is composed of four polypeptide chains, two labeled alpha (α) and two labeled beta (β). Normally, an individual has two normal β genes and four normal α genes. If genes are regulated correctly during replication, approximately equal numbers of α and β globin chains are produced. Each of these globin chains is associated with a heme group, which contains an iron atom that binds with oxygen. This hemoglobin molecule performs the vital function of transporting oxygen in RBCs to organs and structures throughout the body. If the process of replication of RBCs is altered at any step, abnormalities in hemoglobin are the result. The substitution of amino acid with glutamic acid on chromosome 11 at position 6 of the β-globin chain is responsible for SCD (Mankad, 1995).

The composition of normal adult hemoglobin is more than 95 percent hemoglobin A, 1.5–3.5 percent hemoglobin A2, and no hemoglobin S, F, or C. The genotype or genetic makeup of the more common types of SCD is classified as follows according to the Centers for Disease Control and Prevention, as reported by Platt et al. (1984, p. 8):

SS disease: S, F, A2 (<4 percent)

SC disease: S, C

$S\beta^+$ thalassemia: S, F, A, A2

$S\beta^0$ thalassemia: S, F, A2 ($\geq$4 percent)

Current nomenclature includes adding the prefix *SCD* before certain genotypes, such as SCD-SS and SCD-SC (Pass et al., 2000). In homozygous disease (SCD-SS), the genetic makeup consists of two identical abnormal genes.

Numerous permutations are possible during production or replication of the α and β genes. Thalassemia, a group of conditions in which hemoglobin is structurally normal but reduced in quantity, is the second most common hemoglobin disorder worldwide. Heterozygous disease, or sickle cell trait (SA), which is not classified as a type of SCD, generally does not cause clinical symptoms because the majority of hemoglobin is normal (A). Hereditary persistence of fetal hemoglobin (HPFH), likewise, is not classified as SCD; yet HPFH has demonstrated some benefit in individuals with SCD.

Four distinct haplotypes (unit of genes on a single chromosome) originated independently in four different geographic areas—southeastern West Africa (Benin and Senegal), central Africa (Banku), and India (Arab-India). The gene for SCD was brought to the Americas in the hulls of slave ships. Central and southeastern West Africa served as the main source for these slaves. Large numbers of African Americans affected with SCD are still today geographically clustered in areas close to the ports of entry for slave ships. Moreover, individuals in the United States are able to trace their ancestry directly to the family's tribe of origin in Africa by comparing haplotypes in the blood (Edelstein, 1986; Serjeant & Serjeant, 2001; Wailoo, 1997).

The expression of the disease, or phenotype, of the person varies greatly, evidenced by the array of symptoms and complications experienced over the lifetime of individuals. This phenomenon still puzzles scientists, and research continues to seek answers to why severity of disease differs so greatly among individuals with the same genotype, even within the same family.

Transmission

Sickle cell disease is inherited as an autosomal recessive trait, meaning an offspring must receive one abnormal hemoglobin gene from each parent to have the condition. Figure 3.1 illustrates the risks of producing a child with SCD based on the genotype of both parents. With each pregnancy, the odds are the same for producing offspring with any of the possible genotypes. If both parents have sickle cell trait (SA or AS) (Generation I), there is a:

25 percent chance that offspring will have SCD-SS

25 percent chance that offspring will have normal hemoglobin AA

50 percent chance that offspring will have sickle cell trait (Generation II)

Figure 3.1
Transmission of Sickle Cell Disease

<u>Generation</u>

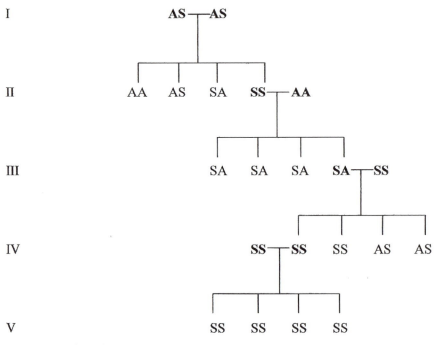

Note: SA and AS are the same.

If one parent has normal hemoglobin and one parent has SCD (II), all off-spring will have sickle cell trait (Generation III). If one parent has sickle cell trait and one parent has SCD (III), the odds are 50 percent that offspring will have SCD and 50 percent that offspring will have sickle cell trait (Generation IV). If both parents have SCD, all offspring will have SCD (Generation V). Figure 3.1 illustrates the importance of African American men and women knowing their sickle cell status in order to make informed reproductive decisions.

Diagnosis

The purpose of testing for SCD is to identify the genotype in at-risk populations or persons presenting with symptoms of SCD so that diagnosis is confirmed, appropriate clinical management instituted, and genetic counseling services offered. Focused research is conducted for reasons such as establishing predictors of severity of disease and discovering more effective treatments.

Laboratory Testing

Options for diagnostic testing include tests that (1) analyze hemoglobin to detect abnormal hemoglobin S; (2) describe red blood cell characteristics; or (3) involve genetic studies. All available tests to diagnose SCD will not be detailed here. In general, a blood specimen is taken. The sickling (slide) or solubility test may be the initial screening method. If this test is positive, the results must be confirmed by hemoglobin electrophoresis. In many instances, further confirmatory testing is conducted. Although not definitive, family studies are inexpensive and are useful in confirming the presence of sickle cell trait and/or disease in a family through careful and detailed history taking from reliable source persons. The most technologically advanced testing is DNA analysis. The expense and need for special equipment and trained technicians, however, makes DNA analysis unfeasible in many settings.

Newborn Screening

In 1987 the National Institutes of Health (NIH) Consensus Development Conference issued its report, *Newborn Screening for Sickle Cell Disease and Other Hemoglobinopathies*, which recommended testing for SCD in all newborns. The purpose of screening newborns is to identify affected infants so as to allow early diagnosis and treatment. Hemoglobin electrophoresis with cellulose acetate is the preferred initial screening tool and is more reliable than other methods for newborns. Most states, however, continue to use filter paper samples. Today testing is universal in 44 of the 50 states, the District of Columbia, Puerto Rico, and the Virgin Islands (National Institutes of Health [NIH], 2002). Screening is available by request in the other six states. All high-risk infants should be tested, meaning those of African, Mediterranean, Middle Easter, Indian, Caribbean, and South and Central American ancestry. Early identification has demonstrated effectiveness in reducing morbidity and mortality of children with SCD because of early intervention, parental education, and penicillin prophylaxis (Wong et al., 1995).

Pathophysiology

The normal red blood cell (RBC) lives 120 days. It is disc shaped and soft, and RBCs flow easily in small blood vessels. Sickle cells are irregularly shaped and hard, and often get stuck in small blood vessels; they live only 20 days or less. Sickle cells are changed by a process known as polymerization, where a portion of the cell wall is removed, leaving that area open and sticky. The sickle cells eventually clump together, causing a blockage in small blood vessels that disrupts the flow of blood (see Figure 3.2). This vaso-occlusive process causes

Figure 3.2
Sickling of Red Blood Cells

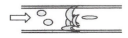

damage to tissues and organs by depriving them of oxygen, which is vital for proper functioning and survival. The lack of adequate oxygen to the tissues and organs causes pain and can lead to temporary or permanent damage to those structures.

Physical Manifestations and Complications

Clinical symptoms are widely variable, and the occurrence of complications in individuals with SCD is highly unpredictable. Almost no organ system is spared. Infection and vaso-occlusive or painful episodes are of the greatest concern. Infections were the leading cause of death in children under the age of two years (Wong et al., 1995) before penicillin prophylaxis was instituted as a major component in standard treatment and management protocols. Table 3.1 lists the most

Table 3.1
Complications of SCD

Body System	Complication
Musculoskeletal	Dactylitis or hand-foot-syndrome in infancy Necrosis of hip and osteomyelitis
Lungs	Acute chest syndrome resulting in chronic lung disease
Abdomen	Splenic sequestration or "bleeding into the spleen" leading to removal of spleen (splenectomy) Gall stones leading to removal of gall bladder (cholecystectomy)
Blood	Chronic anemia causing easy fatigability Aplastic anemia leading to fatal cessation of blood forming process Transfusions that put individuals at-risk for blood-borne infectious diseases, such as HIV/AIDS and hepatitis B & C
Kidney	Chronic kidney failure necessitating hemodialysis
Heart	Congestive heart failure
Neurological	Cerebral vascular accident or stroke Mini-infarcts causing cognitive deficits and learning disabilities
Eyes	Sickle cell retinopathy leading to blindness
Ears	Sensorineural hearing loss
Skin	Chronic leg ulcers
Genitourinary	Priapism or painful penile erection leading to sterility
General	Vaso-occlusion causing acute and chronic pain Fever in children

common complications of SCD (Bloom, 1995; Serjeant & Serjeant, 2001). Pain is the most predominant complication, especially in adults.

Delayed growth is almost universal in children with SCD. These children generally have normal weight and length at birth but experience delayed skeletal growth through puberty. Most eventually do achieve normal or near-normal adult height, if not weight. Research suggests that nutrition plays a role in these developmental delays (Rodgers, 1997). Fertility, however, is likely to be normal by the age of twenty years. These physical manifestations and complications of SCD do occur throughout the life span and often become chronic instead of acute as the individual ages.

One myth to dispel is the belief that sickle cell trait turns into SCD. Unless someone's genetic makeup is altered, this is impossible. Individuals with sickle cell trait do not experience vaso-occlusive symptoms under normal conditions, and they have a normal life expectancy. They can, however, develop microscopic damage to the kidneys and experience hematuria or blood in the urine, which is usually not visible to the naked eye. Women with sickle cell trait have a higher propensity than racially matched controls, especially during pregnancy, to have frequent urinary tract infections (NIH, 2002). There is no contraindication to participation in competitive sports for the person with sickle cell trait. Exercise-related death in individuals with sickle cell trait is more likely a function of an individual not being as physically fit as needed before participating in strenuous physical activity versus being caused by the sickle cell trait status. Risks associated with anesthesia and surgery are not increased either, so there are no special precautions before these procedures or any other health-related matters.

With SCD, physical symptoms are more observable and recognizable. But the emotional impact of SCD can be equally challenging. Researchers have studied psychosocial-biological influences and manifestations in affected individuals from infancy to adulthood.

Psychosocial Implications

Because SCD is an inherited chronic disorder customarily diagnosed at birth, the impact places additional stress on the family unit very early. The knowledge that they have passed abnormal genes to their child can create feelings of guilt, disbelief, anger, fear, and helplessness in parents (Hurtig, 1994). In the past, these parents were not given much hope of survival for their child beyond a few years. Even with extended life expectancy today, given the uncertainty and unpredictability of SCD, the family is still in a vulnerable state. The family's capacity to provide emotional support, as well as care for physical needs, is crucial in helping children develop positive feelings about themselves.

Infants and children up to 4 years old with SCD who are separated from the family for frequent hospitalizations may have difficulties developing trust. Because their thinking is very imaginary, children 4 to 6 years of age may believe their illness is a punishment for something they did and feel a sense of guilt. They may show signs of regression and dependency when they are hospitalized. Overprotective parents and restrictive hospitalizations may oppress the child's first drive for independence. The older child, between 6 and 12 years, is more prone than younger children to display learning delays, secondary to frequent absences from school caused by complications of SCD. The separation from peers may lead to feelings of low self-esteem.

During adolescence, ages 12 to 18 years, the effects of SCD complications become chronic and not just acute episodic occurrences, interfering with the ability to keep up with peers in school academics and physical activity. Delayed sexual development may cause poor body image. These factors combined have a major impact on emotional development and may lead to poor self-esteem, minimal achievement, and limited social success. Adolescents without chronic conditions have conflicts over identity; completing this developmental milestone can be complicated in adolescents with SCD by negative images of their bodies, depression, anxiety, and preoccupation with illness and death. Normal adolescent acting-out behaviors may become a real challenge for the family. A delicate balance between overprotection and encouraging independence must be found. Transition to adult care settings contributes additional stress as the child and parent prepare to leave the safe haven provided by trusted pediatric caregivers (Holbrook & Phillips, 1994; Treadwell & Gil, 1994).

The young adult years of 18 to 35 present the developmental challenge of establishing intimacy, which must be preceded by self-awareness of one's sexuality and acceptance of self and body. This period is customarily the time when most people find mates and marry. Delayed sexual maturation may cause ambivalence for some young adults. Chronic symptoms from complications may interfere with one's ability to maintain employment, fulfill family responsibilities, sustain relationships, and manage one's own health. Depression often occurs. A supportive network (personal and professional) can help these adults with SCD prevent their disease from taking control of their lives or crippling them because of the unpredictability of SCD. Despite these influences, many people do well: they complete college, begin productive careers, and establish their own families. Independence is influenced by relationships within their family, past experiences, knowledge of their disease, severity of the disease, and their general emotional maturity. As they continue to age, diligent self-management and appropriate medical management will allow them to thrive. Many survive well into their 60s and 70s, leading full, normal lives.

African American mothers play a vital role in helping children affected by SCD progress through normal developmental milestones, as well as cope with the added stressors related to chronic illness. The mother becomes, by necessity, an advocate for access to high-quality health care for her child, including mental health services when indicated. If she herself is also affected by SCD, these issues are compounded.

THERAPY FOR SCD

Medical

The most appropriate care for patients with SCD is through a multidisciplinary team consisting of hematologists, doctors specially trained in diseases of the blood; family physicians (or pediatricians for children, internists for adults); obstetrician-gynecologists for women; and nurses, nurse practitioners, and physician assistants. Others may participate in helping the individual and/or family manage responses to the disease: nutritionists, chaplains, psychologists, social workers, and genetic counselors. Medical specialists that can be involved in the care depending on the need are urologists, nephrologists, general and orthopedic surgeons, emergency medicine specialists, anesthesia and pain specialists, and physical and vocational rehabilitation specialists (Platt & Sacerdote, 2002).

Medical care is rendered in a variety of settings, from the physician's private office to primary care clinics, dedicated sickle cell centers, and emergency rooms. Although an important factor in the quality of care provided is the knowledge and experience with SCD of the physician and others on the multidisciplinary team, the most comprehensive care is available in a dedicated sickle cell center. The National Institutes of Health funds ten such centers in different geographic locations on five-year cycles. The current centers are located in the following cities: Bronx and New York, N.Y.; two in Philadelphia, Pa.; Birmingham and Mobile, Ala.; Los Angeles and San Francisco, Calif.; Cincinnati, Ohio; and Boston, Mass.

Insurance coverage for medical care can present challenges for persons affected with SCD. Coverage varies from institution to institution and from state to state. But there is always medical insurance available for persons with SCD due to the chronic nature of the disease. Most individuals without insurance will qualify for social security and federal- and state-funded supplemental programs. It is important that all persons with SCD gain access to health care through some form of insurance coverage because costs can be astronomical due to frequent medical visits, follow-up care, medications, emergency room visits, special testing and procedures, and admissions to hospitals. Keeping informed about health care options is a necessity for persons with SCD in order to maintain appropriate health care.

Standard protocol in the management of individuals with SCD includes a wide gamut of tests and procedures. Medication varies from preventive vaccinations to the therapeutic management of pain. Infants receive the usual vaccinations included in the recommended schedule for childhood immunizations; but they receive the pneumococcal vaccine earlier than their healthy counterparts. All children are prescribed penicillin prophylaxis from birth to five years of age; folic acid supplementation is recommended throughout the life span of the person. Routine blood tests, such as a complete blood count with differential and reticulocyte (red blood cell) count, plus a urinanalysis should be monitored regularly to identify any changes that will alert health care providers to the impending onset of acute illness. Other diagnostics tests are ordered as indicated by any significant presenting symptoms.

Different types of transfusion protocols are reserved for treating severe anemia with hemodynamic compromise, acute vaso-occlusive events that do not respond to conventional therapy, and for the prevention and treatment of stroke. Posttransfusion monitoring of blood levels is critical in the assessment of posttransfusion complications, such as iron overload and congestive heart failure, and to determine if desired blood levels have been reached.

Medications

Pain medication is of primary importance for the person with SCD in that pain is the hallmark symptom of the disease. There are variant degrees of pain medication for mild to severe pain. Accordingly, over-the-counter medications (Tylenol and Motrin) or narcotic analgesics (morphine and dilaudid) are prescribed. Adjuvant medications for the management of chronic, neuropathic, muscular, and psychological pain (antidepressants, anticonvulsants, clonidine, sedatives, antihistamines) are also used. Many individuals with SCD learn to manage pain at home under the direction of a prescribing physician and regulate their pain medication for simple vaso-occlusive crises that have no other complication (NIH, 2002).

Hydroxyurea is a substance that assists the body in producing hemoglobin F, which helps decrease the frequency of acute vaso-occlusive crisis by limiting the sickling process in the cells, and thus improving the quality of life in many individuals with SCD. In the normal infant, high concentrations of hemoglobin F steadily decrease while hemoglobin A increases. By 4 to 6 months of age, the concentration of hemoglobin F is essentially undetectable. In the normal infant, this presents no clinical problems. On the other hand, this sudden change in hemoglobin in an infant with SCD might result in the early manifestation of symptoms associated with the diagnosis of SCD. Individuals with SCD who also have hereditary persistence of hemoglobin F have demonstrated less severe disease over their life span. Thus, hydroxyurea has demonstrated benefit in persons with SCD by stimulating production of hemoglobin F (which has some of the same molecular properties as hemoglobin A). Careful monitoring of individual responses to therapy is mandatory due to potentially adverse side effects of hydroxyurea (NIH, 2002).

Nonmedical

Nonmedical therapy is available for the management of pain for the person with SCD. Such integrative therapies include, but are not limited to, therapeutic touch, imagery, relaxation, distraction techniques, massage, and transcutaneous electric nerve stimulation (TENS). These interventions are effective alone or in conjunction with traditional medical management and are incorporated in the treatment plan in hopes of changing the individual's perception and attitude about health, resulting in actual positive changes in personal behaviors that ultimately promote healing and sustained health (Shames, 1996).

Preventive Care

The goal for the individual with SCD is to maintain wellness by actively engaging in behaviors that promote health and prevent precipitating factors that might lead to severe, acute crises. Guardians, children, and young adults personally or indirectly affected by SCD are taught measures to self-manage the disease. Platt and Sacerdote (2002) created a useful acronym of the basic principles of prevention, called FARMS (p. 45):

F—Fluids and Fever

A—Air

R—Rest

M—Medication and Medical Care

S—Situations to Avoid

Individuals with SCD must drink plenty of water to prevent dehydration, which may cause further sickling. Managing fever from its onset is important, and medical attention must be sought immediately to rule out acute infection. Adequate oxygen intake is critical for the proper functioning of red blood cells, and individuals with SCD are encouraged to get sufficient amounts by breathing fresh air outside and maintaining clean air indoors. Situations that will deprive one of oxygen should be avoided, such as smoking, excessive exercise, or flying in an unpressurized airplane. An individual with SCD may need more rest than a person without SCD. Knowing one's limits and setting realistic expectations for activity are essential to prevent complications. Preventive and therapeutic medications should be taken as prescribed by the health care provider.

Medical care should be sought at the first signs of fever, chest pain, shortness of breath, unusual headache, sudden weakness or loss of feeling, pain that will not subside with home regimen, priapism that does not resolve, or sudden vision changes. Other situations to avoid to maintain health include not getting too hot or too cold (dressing in layers when it is cold and in cool clothing when it is hot, using air conditioning whenever possible), alcohol or illegal drugs, and stress.

Sickle cell disease requires aggressive management throughout the life span of the individual. Cooperation between the individual, the family and the health care team can improve the quality of life and increase the life expectancy of the individual with SCD. Given the appropriate health regimen, the individual can maintain wellness at home and will be more aware of their body and signs and symptoms that may lead to a life-threatening complication. Women with SCD additionally have unique health concerns related to their bodies and reproductive issues.

WOMEN WITH SCD

General Health

The general health of women with SCD is compromised and presents many challenges to the individual. Affecting every body system, the onset of puberty and menarche is delayed in girls with an associated delay in the development of secondary sexual characteristics. This delay was greater in SCD-SS disease and $S\beta^0$ thalassemia than in SCD-SC disease and $S\beta^+$ thalassemia. Weight was the best predictor of menarche, followed by age (Platt et al., 1984). Serjeant and Serjeant (2001) cite several studies that report the mean age at menarche at 13.9 years, compared to 12.2 years in normal black controls in Washington, D.C., and at 16.1 years, compared to 13.1 years among normal Jamaican controls. Studies have not supported the statement that females with SCD are relatively infertile.

Delayed pregnancy is most likely a result of slow development of secondary sexual characteristics after menarche, more reserved personality of these girls, and features of the disease that impair their body image and self-esteem, leading to delayed sexual exposure.

Menstruation is often associated with dysmenorrhea or pain during bleeding, irregular cycles, and heavy bleeding. Research does not demonstrate increased incidence of painful vaso-occlusive episodes during menstruation. The additional loss of blood during menstruation may create a temporary further decline in hemoglobin levels, causing increased fatigue secondary to the state of chronic anemia in SCD.

Reproductive Concerns

Contraception

Women with SCD are entitled to contraceptive counseling and management to prevent unwanted pregnancy as much as any other woman. One argument for preparing teenagers for transition to adult care and transferring them to adult settings during the late teens is to increase the likelihood they will receive comprehensive counseling and services related to sexual issues, something not readily available in pediatric settings. Several methods of contraception are safe for women with SCD. In some European countries, the use of oral contraceptives (OCs) is contraindicated for women with SCD. In the United States, SCD does not contraindicate OC use. The mechanism of action for a vaso-occlusive episode differs from that of a thromboembolic event. Hypoxia to cells starts the sickling process, resulting in the clustering of abnormally shaped red blood cells and blockage of vessels or vaso-occlusion. The mechanism of a thromboembolic event is associated with blood-clotting abnormalities and the formation of clotting within the vessel. Oral contraceptives do not cause hypoxia or exacerbate sickling vaso-occlusive crises and are, therefore, prescribed in the United States for women with SCD, provided there are no other risk factors for a thromboembolic event. Other risk factors may include hypertension, smoking, family history of clot formation, and obesity. Women who have a greater propensity for clot formation that might be induced by OC use should not be prescribed OCs, whether they have SCD or not.

Potential adverse effects from OCs for women with SCD are rare, and the benefits of contraception far outweigh the risks associated with pregnancy for these women, so they should not be denied access to an effective contraception. The World Health Organization is in consensus with this position (Contraceptiononline, 1998). Other contraception options are injectables such as depo-medroxyprogesterone (DepoProvera), which is administered once every three months; implants; barrier methods—diaphragm, condom; and sterilization. Intrauterine devices may be associated with uterine bleeding and infection, and thus are not highly recommended for women with SCD (NIH, 2002). Comprehensive counseling and continued support will improve the chances of contraceptive success for women with SCD.

Conception

At puberty and periodically thereafter women with SCD should receive information about the disease, genetic transmission, methods of contraception, prenatal diagnosis, prevention of sexually transmitted disease, and risks associated with pregnancy. Even though sexual maturation may be delayed, most women will catch up to their normal peers and achieve fertility while in their teenage years. Genetic counseling will help them understand the odds of producing offspring with SCD, given the knowledge of the sickle status of their sexual partner. Various genetic tests are available to women who are diagnosed with SCD. These tests can be performed before and after conception to determine the sickle cell status of the unborn fetus. Preimplantation genetic diagnosis is expensive and not readily available everywhere; prenatal diagnosis from in utero sampling is more common. Information on this detail can clarify alternatives and help a woman weigh the benefits and risks of pregnancy. Influencing factors will also include the woman's religious, ethical, and moral beliefs and cultural background.

Hydroxyurea has been shown to be teratogenic in animal models. Therefore, women with SCD who are taking hydroxyurea should stop the medication three to six months before trying to conceive. Likewise, women must be aware that if their sexual partner is a man with SCD who are taking hydroxyurea, he should stop the medication before attempting to impregnate her (Halsey & Roberts, 2003).

Pregnancy Issues

A pregnant woman with SCD is able to carry a fetus to term and deliver a healthy baby with careful management from a multidisciplinary team: a primary care provider, an obstetrician, and a hematologist all familiar with SCD, plus a nutritionist. Counseling is an essential component prior to pregnancy and during the postpartum period. Once the woman with SCD becomes pregnant, there are additional concerns such as infection, frequency of vaso-occlusive crises, hypertension and preeclampsia, spontaneous abortions, stillbirths, and fetal and maternal mortality. If appropriate perinatal care is provided throughout the pregnancy in a high-risk facility, risks for the woman with SCD can be greatly decreased.

Perinatal Care

Throughout the entire pregnancy, the woman needs to be monitored closely for any sudden changes that may precipitate onset of high-risk complications. The prenatal assessment is a crucial part of the management of the pregnancy process for these women. A comprehensive history is recommended to alert health care providers of any additional risk factors that may be imminent or life threatening to mother and fetus. Laboratory studies and a nutritional assessment are an essential part of the prenatal evaluation. The hemoglobin level may steadily decline during pregnancy, most significantly in women with SCD-SS disease. Women should take prenatal vitamins, which contain many minerals and nutrients, in addition to their normal regimen of folic acid supplementation. Anticipated weight gain is similar to that of women without SCD.

During pregnancy, the incidence of common medical problems, such as urinary tract infection, hypertension, and albuminuria, is increased in women with SCD. They also may experience more frequently complications of SCD, particularly acute chest syndrome and bone pain. More frequent visits to health care providers for monitoring of mother and fetus are recommended to prevent or manage complications early.

Delivery poses additional concerns if the woman has pelvic changes secondary to delayed menarche and development of secondary sexual characteristics. Most women, however, are able to have a normal vaginal delivery. After delivery, many women develop elevated temperatures from endometritis and postdelivery wound infection. Postpartum hemorrhage is not increased in these women compared to women without SCD.

With proper care during pregnancy, women with SCD can carry to full term with minimal risk for additional complications as a result of having SCD. Whether the child is diagnosed with SCD or not at birth, there is a good chance that the infant will otherwise be healthy and thrive throughout all stages of life.

FUTURE DIRECTIONS AND RESEARCH

New and innovative treatments and procedures (Bloom, 1995; NIH, 2002; Platt & Sacerdote, 2002) continue to provide hope to the SCD population. Treatments include, but are not limited to, experimental medications, gene therapy, and stem cell transplantation. Current research is directed toward altering the structure of the mutant gene to discover a cure for SCD. Scientists believe that the only true cure for SCD lies in gene therapy. All other treatments are palliative in nature and only treat symptoms, thus preventing the complication that may result if no action is taken. Hydroxyurea and several medications have previously been discussed. Additional experimental medications are being evaluated to determine effectiveness in hydrating red blood cells (RBCs), preventing sickling, increasing hemoglobin F, and decreasing the viscosity of RBCs. These agents demonstrate potential for alleviating the vaso-occlusive process frequently associated with sickle cell crisis.

Gene therapy is the process by which the genetic material of a cell is altered by external manipulation. In SCD, the ultimate aim is to stimulate the production of normal hemoglobin genes at the level of stem cell maturation into healthy RBCs. Many questions about gene therapy and its effectiveness in stopping the mutant gene from producing hemoglobin S and stimulating instead the production of hemoglobin A remain unanswered.

Stem cell transplantation is the process by which bone marrow cells with normal hemoglobin are transplanted into the bone marrow of an individual with abnormal hemoglobin. Appropriate donors are limited because the criteria for matching are very rigorous and related to the genetic similarities between donor and recipient. Siblings usually have very similar genetic material and make suitable donors. Because of the negative risk-versus-benefit ratio associated with bone marrow transplantation in persons with SCD, it is not frequently recommended as a first line of therapy.

Although individuals with SCD, including children, often participate in several research studies concurrently, most are selective and ever hopeful that a cure for SCD will be found during their lifetime or a discovery to directly benefit them. Participant burnout, occurs frequently so researchers must be sensitive to the physical and emotional needs of participants, who already represent a vulnerable population due to the nature of SCD and their African American ethnicity. Dedicated practitioners and researchers strive on in their efforts to make a difference in the lives of individuals with SCD. Sickle cell disease was the first molecular disease described, yet a cure is still elusive.

REFERENCES

Bloom, M. 1995. *Understanding Sickle Cell Disease.* Jackson: University Press of Mississippi.

Bullock, W. H., and P. N. Jilly. 1975. Hematology. In R. A. Williams, *Textbook of Black-related diseases* (pp. 199–316). St. Louis: McGraw-Hill.

Chestnut, D. E. 1994. Perceptions of ethnic and cultural factors in the delivery of services in the treatment of sickle cell disease. In R. B. Nash (Ed.), *Psychosocial Aspects of Sickle Cell Disease: Past, Present and Future Directions of Research* (pp. 215–242). New York: Haworth Press.

Contraceptiononline. 1998. Oral contraceptives and sickle cell disease. *The Contraceptive Report,* 8(6):9–11. Accessed August 12, 2004, at http://www.contraceptiononline.org/contrareport/previssues.cfm.

Edelstein, S. J. 1986. *The Sickled Cell: From Myths to Molecules.* Cambridge, MA: Harvard University Press.

Feldman, S. D., and A. I. Tauber. 1997. Sickle cell anemia: Reexamining the first "molecular disease." *Bulletin of the History of Medicine,* 71, 623–650.

Halsey, C., and I.A.G. Roberts. 2003. The role of hydroxyurea in sickle cell disease. *British Journal of Haematology,* 120, 177–186.

Herrick, J. B. 1910. Peculiar elongated and sickle-shaped red blood corpuscles in a case of severe anemia. *Archives of Internal Medicine,* 6, 517–521.

Holbrook, C. T., and G. Phillips. 1994. Natural history of sickle cell disease and the effects on biopsychosocial development. In R. B. Nash (Ed.), *Psychosocial Aspects of Sickle Cell Disease: Past, Present, and Future Directions in Research* (pp. 7–18). New York: Haworth Press.

Hurtig, A. L. 1994. Relationships in families of children and adolescents with sickle cell disease. In R. B. Nash (Ed.), *Psychsocial Aspects of Sickle Cell Disease: Past, Present, and Future Directions in Research* (pp. 161–183). New York: Haworth Press.

Lebby, R. 1846. Case of absence of the spleen. *Southern Journal of Medicine and Pharmacy,* 1, 481–483.

Lessin, L. S., and W. N. Jensen. 1974. Sickle cell anemia 1910–1973: An overview. *Archives of Internal Medicine,* 133, 529–532.

Mankard, V. N. 1995. Sickle cell disease and other disorders of abnormal hemoglobin. In D. R. Miller (Ed.), *Blood Diseases of Infancy and Childhood: In the Tradition of Carl H. Smith* (pp. 415–459). St. Louis: Mosby.

National Institutes of Health, National Heart, Lung, and Blood Institute. 2002. *The Management of Sickle Cell Disease.* NIH Pub. No. 02-2117. Bethesda, MD: U.S. Department of Health and Human Services.

National Sickle Cell Anemia Control Act. 1972. In *United States Statutes at Large,* 86, 137 [P. L. 92-294]. Washington, D.C.: Government Printing Office.

NIH Consensus Development Conference Statement. 1987. Newborn screening for sickle cell disease and other hemoglobinopathies. *NIH Consensus Statement,* 6(9): 1–22. Available at http://consensus.nih.gov/1987/1987ScreeningSickleHemoglobinopat hies061html.htm.

Pass, K. A., P. A. Lane, P. M. Fernhoff, C. F. Hinton, S. R. Panny, J. S. Parks., et al. 2000. U.S. newborn screening system guidelines II: follow-up of children, diagnosis, management, and evaluation. Statement of the Council of Regional Networks for Genetic Services. *Journal of Pediatrics,* 137(Suppl. 4):S1–46.

Pauling, L., H. Itana, S. J. Singer, and I. C. Wells. 1949. Sickle cell anemia: A molecular disease. *Science,* 110, 543–548.

Platt, A. F., and A. Sacerdote. 2002. *Hope and Destiny: The Patient's and Parent's Guide to Sickle Cell Disease and Sickle Cell Trait.* Roscoe, IL: Hilton Publishing Company.

Platt, O. S., D. J. Brambilla, W. F. Rosse, P. F. Milner, O. Castro, M. Steinberg, et al. 1994. Mortality in sickle cell disease: Life expectancy and risk factors for early death. *The New England Journal of Medicine,* 330, 1639–1644.

Platt, O. S., W. Rosenstock, and M. A. Espeland. 1984. Influence of sickle hemoglobinopathies on growth and development. *The New England Journal of Medicine,* 311, 7–12.

Rodgers, G. P. 1997. Overview of pathophysiology and rationale for treatment of sickle cell anemia. *Seminars in Hematology,* 34(Suppl. 3):2–7.

Serjeant, G. R., and B. E. Serjeant. 2001. *Sickle Cell Disease* (3rd ed.). New York: Oxford University Press.

Shames, K. H. 1996. Harness the power of guided imagery. *RN,* 59(8):49–50.

Treadwell, M. J., and K. M. Gil. 1994. Psychosocial aspects. In S. H. Embury, R. P. Hebbel, N. Mohandas, and M. H. Steinberg (Eds.), *Sickle Cell Disease: Basic Principles and Clinical Practice* (pp. 517–529). New York: Raven Press.

Wailoo, K. 1991. "A disease *sui generi*": The origins of sickle cell anemia and the emergence of modern clinical research, 1904–1924. *Bulletin of the History of Medicine,* 65, 185–208.

———. 1997. *Drawing Blood: Technology and Disease Identity in Twentieth-Century America.* Baltimore, MD: Johns Hopkins University Press.

Whitten, C. F., and J. Fischhoff. 1974. Psychosocial effects of sickle cell disease. *Archives of Internal Medicine,* 133, 681–689.

Williams-Morris, R. S. 1996. Racism and children's health: Issues in development. *Ethnicity and Disease,* 6(1–2):69–82.

Wong, W. Y., D. R. Powars, and G. D. Overturf. 1995. Infections in children with sickle cell anemia. *Infectious Medicine,* 12, 331–338.

4

Sickle Cell Disease: What's Going On? Insights for Women

CHERYL HUNTER-GRANT

Although Western medicine described sickle cell disease almost hundred years ago, the peoples of Africa have known it for hundreds of years. Many different names have been used by various West African ethnic groups to describe the condition.

Twi tribe: ahotutuo

Faute tribe: nwiiwii

Ewe tribe: nuidudui

Ga tribe: chwechweechwe. (Bridges, 2002)

If sickle cell disease has been "known" for so long, why does the disease still exist? What's going on? The short answer to the latter question would be, "Not enough," since there is still no cure for the disease. The longer answer would be—"A lot!" While there is no cure, significant advances have been made since the early discovery. But there is still much more that can be done. We cannot stop until we have a cure.

SICKLE CELL DISEASE

Sickle cell disease is the category of hematologic (blood) diseases caused when an individual has at least one gene for sickle hemoglobin and one gene for any other unusual hemoglobin, commonly S, C, D, and Thalassemia. An autosomal recessive inherited disease, sickle cell disease is passed from parent to child, affecting about 72,000 Americans predominately of African Ancestry (National Institutes of Health [NIH], 2002b).

Sickle cell disease "is most common in West and Central Africa where as many as 25% of the people have sickle cell trait and 1–2% of all babies are born with a form of the disease. In the United States with an estimated population of over 270 million, about 1,000 babies (1 in 400) are born with sickle cell disease each year. In contrast, in Nigeria, which has an estimated 1997 population of 90 million, 45,000–90,000 babies with sickle cell disease are born each year" (Sickle Cell Disease Association of America, n.d.). One in 12 African Americans has sickle cell trait.

The sickle gene was brought into the Americas and the Caribbean primarily through the slave trade. However, sickle cell disease had already spread from Africa to Southern Europe by the time of the slave trade, so it is present in Portuguese, Spaniards, French Corsicans, Sardinians, Sicilians, mainland Italians, Greeks, Turks, and Cypriots. Sickle cell disease appears in most of the Near and Middle East countries, including Lebanon, Israel, Saudi Arabia, Kuwait and Yemen. The condition has also been reported in India and Sri Lanka.

Sickle cell disease is an international health problem and truly a global challenge. All these countries must work together to solve the problem and find effective treatments and ultimately a cure. The knowledge and expertise in the management of sickle cell disease acquired in the technologically advanced countries must be shared with the less developed countries where patients die at alarming rates. (Sickle Cell Disease Association of America, n.d.)

Sickle cell trait (the carrier state of the sickle gene) developed as a genetic mutation that protected young children from certain forms of malaria. Malaria continues to be a problem in Africa. One million African children still die each year from the illness. Sickle cell trait is still a protective mutation for children in Africa, partially protecting them from the deadly consequences of malaria. In countries where malaria is not endemic, sickle cell trait offers no protective advantage.

Sickle cell anemia (the classic form of sickle cell disease) is characterized by chronic anemia and periodic episodes of pain. Duane R. Bonds, M.D., leader of the sickle cell disease scientific research group at the National Heart, Lung, and Blood Institute (NHLBI), a component of the National Institutes of Health (NIH) located in Bethesda, Md., has characterized the sickle cell blockages or "log jams" that occur in small vessels similar to having "mini heart attacks throughout the entire body. A heart attack is painful because the blood flow to the heart is interrupted. In sickle cell anemia, the blood flow can be interrupted to any of the major organs, causing severe pain and organ damage at the site of the blood flow blockage" (Mayfield, 1999, p. 1).

Sickle cell disease is not communicable, nor does sickle cell *trait* turn into sickle cell *disease*. Sickle cell disease and trait are determined at the point of conception. Every individual inherits a pair of genes, one half from their mother and one half from their father. Genes determine an individual's characteristics such as height, hair color, eye color, hemoglobin type, and so on. When a person

Figure 4.1
Image of Usual Inheritance Pattern for Sickle Cell Anemia—AS $\times$ AS

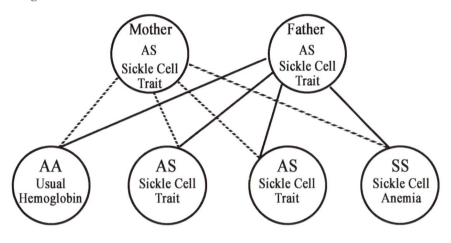

inherits two genes for the usual type of hemoglobin, they are known to have hemoglobin AA.

If a person has inherited one gene for the usual type of hemoglobin (A) and one gene for sickle hemoglobin, known as "S," that person would be known to have sickle cell trait (hemoglobin AS). *Sickle cell trait* is the carrier state of the sickle gene. A person who has sickle cell trait or sickle cell disease can pass their sickle gene on to their children. Generally people who have sickle cell trait are not sick and may not be aware of their trait status without special blood tests that determine hemoglobin type (i.e., hemoglobin electrophoresis).

When a person inherits the sickle (S) gene from both parents, they have sickle cell anemia (hemoglobin SS), the classic form of sickle cell disease. If a person inherits the sickle (S) gene from one parent and another unusual hemoglobin gene such as hemoglobin C from the other parent, they also have sickle cell disease. This particular type is known as hemoglobin SC disease.

The usual inheritance pattern for persons who have sickle cell anemia is having two parents who have sickle cell trait (see Figure 4.1). The usual inheritance pattern for an individual who has hemoglobin SC disease is found in Figure 4.2. One parent has sickle cell trait and one parent has hemoglobin C trait.

To learn the risk of having a child with sickle cell disease, people should be tested to determine their hemoglobin type. The hemoglobin electrophoresis is one of the most accurate tests available for determining hemoglobin type. Genetic counseling, providing nondirective information about the inheritance patterns, origins and implications of the hemoglobin gene; the difference between sickle cell and other hemoglobin traits and sickle cell disease; and health problems that can occur; should be sought (New York State Department of Health, 2002). Counseling should be provided by a specially trained health educator, master's trained genetic counselor or others with training in counseling for sickle cell.

Figure 4.2
Image of Usual Inheritance Pattern for Hemoglobin Sickle Cell Disease—AS × AC

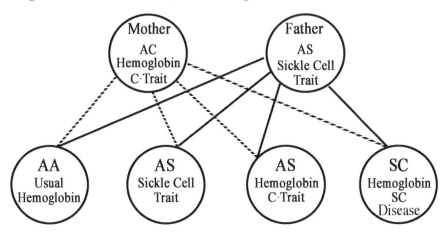

SYMPTOMS AND COMPLICATIONS OF SICKLE CELL DISEASE

The primary job of hemoglobin is to deliver oxygen throughout the body. The alteration present in sickle hemoglobin causes the cell, which is usually a round, disk-like shape, to morph into a sickle-like shape when oxygen is released. Unlike normal red blood cells, which are flexible and pliable, sickle cells are rigid and fragile, creating blockages in blood vessels preventing the flow of blood. Normal red blood cells can live in the blood stream about 120 days. Sickle red blood cells live only about 10–20 days. Since the body cannot replace these cells fast enough, the blood is chronically short of red blood cells, causing anemia.

Since blood flows throughout the entire body, the impact of this sickling process can cause complications throughout the body. Common symptoms and complications of sickle cell disease include: *hand-foot syndrome, or dactylitis,* swelling and pain caused by small vessel blockages in the hands and/or feet that may occur along with fever. This may be the first symptom of sickle cell anemia in infants. Another is *painful episodes or vaso-occulusive episodes,* unpredictable pain that occurs in the bones, joints, and organs due to sickle blood cells blocking oxygen flow to tissues. The frequency and amount of pain can vary and can be acute, chronic or both. The pain may last for only a few hours or as long as several weeks. This condition may require hospitalization and treatment with painkillers and intravenous fluids. This is the most common symptom of sickle cell disease in both children and adults.

Moreover, *infections* due to repeated episodes of sickling in the spleen result in damage that compromises the spleen's ability to destroy bacteria in the blood. This causes both children and adults to be more prone to infections. Infants and young children are especially susceptible to bacterial infections that can kill them in as few as nine hours from onset of fever. Until their immune system is fully developed, young children rely on a properly functioning spleen to filter out damaged cells and bacteria from their blood. Pneumococcal infections used to be the principal cause of death in children with sickle cell anemia until physicians began routinely giving penicillin on a preventive basis to those who are diagnosed at birth or in early infancy. Pneumococcal vaccines are also administered to reduce the risk of obtaining these infections.

Sickling in the small blood vessels in the brain can also lead to serious, life-threatening *strokes*, primarily in children. Even if they survive, children may be left with partial paralysis and/or other neurological impairments. Trapping of red blood cells into the spleen causing a rapid decrease in hemoglobin level called *acute splenic sequestration* is another complication of sickle cell disease. This condition remains the leading cause of death in young children who have sickle cell disease. Pain in the chest caused by infection or trapped sickled cells in the lung, *acute chest syndrome*, can also be a life-threatening complication of sickle cell disease.

Other non-life threatening symptoms of the disease include: *fatigue, paleness, and shortness of breath*, symptoms of the chronic anemia or a shortage of red blood cells; and *jaundice*, the yellowing of skin and eyes resulting from rapid breakdown of red blood cells. Additionally, many individuals who have sickle cell disease may experience a *delay in growth and sexual maturation*. This is primarily caused from a shortage of red blood cells. Typically individuals will catch up to their peers in time. Males who have sickle cell disease may experience *priapism*, a painful uncontrollable erection of the penis caused by blood flow blockage, which may happen episodically, chronically or both. *Leg ulcers*, open sores above and around the ankle area are another common symptom of the disease. Some ulcers heal quickly; others may not heal, and can become painful and recurrent. Sickling of cells in the kidney can cause blood to appear in the urine, a condition known as *hematuria*. Additionally, *eye problems* affecting the retina, the area in the back of the eye that receives and processes visual images, can deteriorate when it does not get enough nourishment from circulating red blood cells. Damage to the retina can be serious enough to cause blindness. Over time with repeated episodes of sickling and blood deprivation in the shoulders or hips, a painful, progressive erosion of the bone in the shoulder or hip, *Avascular Necrosis*, can occur. Finally, in recurring episodes of oxygen deprivation to the organs during repetitive vaso-occlusive and other sickling episodes (*organ damage*), organs die slowly over time and can eventually cause death.

The clinical course of sickle cell disease is very variable. Some individuals have mild symptoms and others have very severe symptoms. This variability can exist even among siblings who have sickle cell disease. While there is no cure for sickle cell disease, individuals who are diagnosed early (ideally at birth), receive good medical care from health professionals trained in managing sickle cell disease (ideally in comprehensive sickle cell centers) can live longer more productive lives. Individuals who have sickle cell disease can now live into the seventh and eighth decade of life (NIH, 2002a).

"Living *with* sickle cell disease" is just what many individuals who have the disease and parents of children who have sickle cell disease will tell you need to happen to live a healthy and productive life. Sickle cell disease can be over-whelming at times, so it is important to be well informed and learn as much about the disease as possible. It is also important to know the *"triggers"* that may precipitate a sickle cell painful episode. Early diagnosis of the disease is also an important factor to minimizing the impact of the early symptoms of sickle cell disease.

To reduce the morbidity and mortality associated with the disease, early identification of sickle cell disease in children is critical. In 1986 the NHLBI Penicillin Prophylaxis in Sickle Cell Disease Study led by Dr. Marilyn Gaston, former deputy branch chief of the Sickle Cell Disease Branch, proved con-clusively that young children placed on prophylactic penicillin had significantly lower rates of death from infections, the major cause of death in young children (Gaston et al., 1986). This was the first preventative therapy for children who have sickle cell disease. Based on these findings, an expert panel convened in 1997 by the NIH and chaired by Doris L. Wethers, M.D., former director of St. Luke's-Roosevelt Hospital Comprehensive Sickle Cell Center, recommended screening at birth for sickle cell disease for all infants born in the United States and placing all affected infants on prophylactic penicillin by the age of three months (Consensus Conference, 1987).

Although it has taken a while for states to act upon these recommendations, today most babies in the United States are screened and identified through state newborn screening programs. By 2003, forty-eight states, the District of Col-umbia, Puerto Rico and the Virgin Islands universally were screening every baby for sickle cell disease. Two states, New Hampshire and South Dakota, have not yet implemented universal newborn screening for sickle cell disease. In New Hampshire, screening is offered only for at-risk babies, and it is offered only by request in South Dakota.

According to the 2000 American Academy of Pediatrics (AAP) Newborn Screening Task Force Report, despite the 1987 NIH Consensus Conference recommendations for universal screening, it has taken many states several years to implement the practice. "Concerns about prevalence, cost-effectiveness, as well as concerns about the acceptability of screening to health professionals and the general public" (AAP, 2000) delayed or hindered implementation of the test. While sickle cell disease is the most prevalent condition included in U.S. newborn screening programs, the prevalence within states varies widely. Inter-estingly, the national incidence for other tests, Phenylketonuria (PKU) and Galactosemia (enzyme deficiencies which diagnosed and treated beginning at birth reduces risk of mental retardation and brain damage), which are included in the newborn screening panels for states who delayed or have yet to include universal screening for sickle cell disease in their newborn screening panels, occur with a frequency of 1:13,947 and 1:53,261 respectively, much lower than sickle cell disease, with a frequency of 1:3,721 for sickle cell anemia and of 1:7,386 for Hemoglobin sickle C disease (U.S. General Accounting Office, 2003). "Thus, while an African-American infant born in a state that does not universally screen for sickle cell disease has the same risk for sickle cell disease as an African-American infant born in a state with universal screening for sickle cell disease, the infant born in the non-screening state is denied the important benefit of screening" (American Academy of Pediatrics, 2000, p. 392).

MILESTONES IN SICKLE CELL DISEASE

Significant advances have occurred in the United States regarding our knowledge of sickle cell disease since the early 1900s (see Table 4.1). Some of the milestones, which have improved our understanding and led to enhancements in the clinical management of the disease, include:

1910—James B. Herrick, a Chicago physician, first described sickle cells in a blood sample from a dental student from Grenada. The term "sickle cell anemia" was coined because of his report.

1972–1973—The National Heart, Lung, and Blood Institute (NHLBI) began funding the first fifteen of its Comprehensive Sickle Cell Centers.

1978—The NHLBI began an epidemiological study of the natural history of sickle cell disease. The Cooperative Study of Sickle Cell Disease (CSSCD) included more than 4,000 individuals, ranging in age from newborns to adults in the sixth decade; it was the first multi-institutional study designed to document prospectively the clinical course of sickle cell disease from birth to adulthood.

1986—The NHLBI Penicillin Prophylaxis in Sickle Cell Disease Study reported that infants and young children placed on prophylactic penicillin had significantly lower rated of *Stepococcus pneumoniae* infections than children who received a placebo. The study established the first preventive therapy for children with sickle cell disease and resulted in a significant reduction in the major cause of death in young children.

1987—An expert panel convened by the NIH to discuss newborn screening for sickle cell disease recommended screening at birth for sickle cell disease for all infants born in the United States and placing all affected infants on prophylactic penicillin by the age of three months. Forty-four states, the District of Columbia, Puerto Rico, and the U.S. Virgin Islands presently screen for newborns with sickle cell disease.

1995—The Multicenter Study of Hydroxyurea in Sickle Cell Anemia (MSH) demonstrated the first effective therapy for severely affected adults with sickle cell disease; painful episodes were reduced by 50 percent.

2000—A multicenter group at thirty sites reported that acute chest syndrome (a respiratory complication associated with sickle cell disease) is commonly precipitated by fat embolism and infection, especially community-acquired pneumonia. Adult patients with neurological symptoms frequently developed respiratory failure. Aggressive treatment with transfusions and bronchodilators improved oxygenation and allowed most patients with respiratory failure to recover (NIH, 2002b).

2004—Researchers at the University of Texas Southwestern Medical Center at Dallas, document that children who have sickle cell disease are living longer, dying less often from their disease and contracting fewer fatal infections than ever before (Quinn et al., 2004).

2005—First once-daily oral iron chelator receives FDA approval. Exjade (deferasirox) will be used for the treatment of chronic iron overload due to frequent blood transfusions in adults and children over the age of two years (Novartis, 2005, SCDAA, 2005).

Table 4.1
Milestones in Sickle Cell Disease

1973—Garrick and coworkers developed methods for neonatal screening employing spots of blood on filter paper.	**1997**—The Stroke Prevention Trial in Sickle Cell Anemia (STOP) demonstrated that periodic transfusions could prevent first time stroke in susceptible children.
1974—Pearson and colleagues demonstrated the feasibility of routine screening of all newborns for sickle cell disease.	**2001**—Pawliuk, Leboulch, and colleagues for the first time corrected sickle cell disease in a transgenic mouse model by gene therapy.
1975—New York State is the 1st state to screen all babies for sickle cell disease.	
1996—The first multicenter study of bone marrow transplantation in children with sickle cell disease reported that the procedure can cure young sickle cell patients who have a matched sibling marrow donor.	**2005**—New oral iron chelator holds potential to transform treatment standard for individuals who have sickle cell disease and require frequent transfusions.

HISTORY OF FUNDING

Federal funding for sickle cell disease in the United States began with the National Sickle Cell Anemia Control Act (P.L. 92-294) on May 16, 1972. The law provided for the creation of voluntary sickle cell anemia screening and counseling programs; information and education programs for health professionals and the public; and research and research training in the diagnosis, treatment and control of sickle cell anemia. The National Sickle Cell Program was born and assigned to the NHLBI. Since 1972, the NHLBI has invested $1.37 billion in sickle cell research (NIH, 2002a, 2003, 2005). Although this investment has accomplished a great deal, it still pales in comparison to the need. Many have called sickle cell disease "the forgotten disease."

It is estimated that between 72,000 and 80,000 Americans have sickle cell disease. In FY 2003, NIH spent $95 million on sickle cell research. It spent $98 million in FY 2004, and is projected to spend $91.4 million in FY 2005. In comparison, Cystic Fibrosis (CF), another autosomal recessive inherited disease which primarily affects Caucasians of European ancestry, received $117 million in FY 2003, $120 million in FY 2004 and is projected to receive $122 million in FY 2005 (NIH, 2005). According to the Cystic Fibrosis Foundation, CF affects 30,000 Americans. Sickle Cell Disease affects 145 percent more Americans than Cystic Fibrosis, however CF receives 22 percent more NIH funding annually than sickle cell.

The South Central Pennsylvania Sickle Cell Council believes the limited support of federal dollars for research may partially be explained by the "misperception that sickle cell disease is solely a disease of Americans of known African descent" (South Central Pennsylvania Sickle Cell Council, n.d.). They call for a national campaign that will educate and increase awareness of the widespread prevalence of sickle cell disease in the United States. The former U.S. Surgeon General David Satcher, on a 2001 health documentary aired on the Discovery Channel, also noted the disparity of federal funding between diseases and agreed that sickle cell disease has been forgotten. "Some diseases because of the people they affect and the lobby behind them certainly have gotten more funding than others," Dr. Satcher says. "I don't like to do battle among diseases. I think we ought to be concerned about all of them. But I believe what is needed in this country is more balance. We in this county have not yet developed a health system that meets the needs of all people and our health system leaves too many gaps—wide gaps—in terms of what's available to different people" (CBS News, 2001).

Today the NIH provides funding for ten Comprehensive Sickle Cell Centers (Table 4.2). These centers are comprised of multidisciplinary researchers and other health professionals who must focus on basic and clinical research as well as community service related to sickle cell disease. Behavioral research, laboratory and data analysis, and quality service activities including diagnosis, education, and counseling are also hallmarks of the Comprehensive Sickle Cell Centers. The centers currently funded are: Boston Comprehensive Sickle Cell Center, Bronx Comprehensive Sickle Cell Center, Children's Hospital of Philadelphia Comprehensive Sickle Cell Center, Cincinnati Comprehensive Sickle Cell Center, Duke-UNC Comprehensive Sickle Cell Center, Marian Anderson Comprehensive Sickle Cell Center, Northern California Comprehensive Sickle Cell Center, St. Jude Children's Research Hospital Comprehensive Sickle Cell Center, Southwestern Comprehensive Sickle Cell Center, and University of Southern California Comprehensive Sickle Cell Center (contact information can be found at the end of this chapter.)

The NIH has primary responsibility for disease research. To meet the public health needs of sickle cell disease, the NIH transferred funding to the Health Resources and Services Administration's (HRSA) Maternal and Child Health Bureau (MCHB) under the 1972 Sickle Cell Disease Act and the subsequent 1978 National Genetic Disease Act (Title XI of the Public Health Service Act). These funds were to be used to develop community-based sickle cell education, screening and counseling services. Since 1972, HRSA has spent approximately $82 million on sickle cell programs.

A significant portion of HRSA's resources has been spent in the area of newborn screening for sickle cell disease. Although there is no cure for sickle cell disease, research has proven that early diagnosis and treatment of the disease, including the administration of prophylactic penicillin, significantly reduces the risk of early mortality and morbidity.

For the past several years (2002–2005), HRSA has provided $10.9 million in funding to improve state sickle cell disease and newborn screening programs (HRSA, 2002, 2003, 2005). In 2003, 17 two-year grants were awarded and in 2005, 18 awards were made for projects which will "link state newborn screening programs, comprehensive sickle cell treatment centers and health care professionals with community-based organizations to provide services" (HRSA, 2003, 2005). The Sickle Cell Disease Association of America, a national

Table 4.2

List of Comprehensive Sickle Cell Centers and Additional Resources

Comprehensive Sickle Cell Centers

Boston Medical Center Comprehensive Sickle Cell Center
Director—Martin Steinberg, M.D.
One Boston Medical Center Place, FGH-2
Boston, MA 02118
617-414-1020 fax 617-414-1021
msteinberg@medicine.bumc.bu.edu

Bronx Comprehensive Sickle Cell Center
Director—Ronald L. Nagel, M.D.
Albert Einstein College of Medicine
Division of Hematology
Ullman Building, Room 921
1300 Morris Park Avenue
Bronx, NY 10461
718-430-2088 fax 718-824-3153
nagel@aecom.yu.edu

Children's Hospital of Philadelphia Comprehensive Sickle Cell Center
Director—Kwaku Ohene-Frempong, M.D.
34th Street & Civic Center Blvd.
Philadelphia, PA 19104
215-590-3423 fax 215-590-2499
ohene-frempong@email.chop.edu

Cincinnati Comprehensive Sickle Cell Center
Director—Clinton H. Joiner, M.D., Ph.D.
Children's Hospital Medical Center
Division of Hematology/Oncology
3333 Burnet Avenue
Cincinnati, OH 45229-3039
513-636-4541 fax 513-636-5562
clint.joiner@chmcc.org

Duke-UNC Comprehensive Sickle Cell Center
Director—Marilyn Telen, M.D.
Division of Hematology
Box 2615
Duke University Medical Center
Durham, NC 27710
919-684-5378 fax 919-681-7688
telen002@mc.duke.edu

Marian Anderson Sickle Cell Anemia Care and Research Center
Director—Marie J. Stuart, M.D.
Thomas Jefferson University
Hematology Division, Pediatrics Dept.
College Bldg., Suite 727
1025 Walnut Street
Philadelphia, PA 19107
215-955-9820 fax 215-955-8011
marie.stuart@mail.tju.edu

Northern California Comprehensive Sickle Cell Center
Director—Elliott Vichinsky, M.D.
Children's Hospital & Research at Oakland
Dept. of Hematology/Oncology
747 52nd Street
Oakland, CA 94609
510-428-3651 fax 510-450-5647
evichinsky@mail.cho.org

St. Jude Children's Research Hospital Comprehensive Sickle Cell Center
Director—Winfred Wang, M.D.
St. Jude Children's Research Hospital
Department of Hematology/Oncology
332 North Lauderdale Bldg, R-6010
Mail Stop Code 763
Memphis, TN 38105
901-495-3497 fax 901-495-2952
Winfred.Wang@stjude.org

Southwestern Comprehensive Sickle Cell Center
Director—George Buchanan, M.D.
The University of Texas
Southwestern Medical Center at Dallas
Pediatrics Department
5323 Harry Hines Boulevard
Dallas, TX 75390-9063
214-648-8594 fax 214-648-3122
George.Buchanan@UTSouthwestern.edu

Comprehensive Sickle Cell Centers (*Continued*)

University of Southern California Comprehensive Sickle Cell Center
Director—Cage S. Johnson, M.D.
Department of Medicine
RMR 304
2025 Zonal Avenue
Los Angeles, CA 90033
323-442-1259 fax 323-442-1255
cagejohn@hsc.usc.edu

Additional Resources

Sickle Cell Disease Association of America, Inc.
200 Corporate Pointe, Suite 495
Culver City, CA 90230-8727
Phone: 310-216-6363
Fax: 310-215-3722
Toll Free: 800-421-8453
http://sicklecelldisease.org/
E-mail: scdaa@sicklecelldisease.org

Sickle Cell Advisory Consortium, Inc. (SCAC)
c/o Brookdale University Hospital
& Medical Center
Comprehensive Sickle Cell Program
One Brookdale Plaza—Suite 346 CHC
Brooklyn, NY 11212
Phone: 718-240-5904
Fax: 718-240-6730
E-mail: SCAConsortium@hotmail.com

SCAC Guidelines for the Treatment of People with Sickle Cell Disease
(March 2002) http://www.wadsworth.org/
newborn/scellguidelines.pdf

The South Central Pennsylvania Sickle Cell Council
3211 North Front Street, Suite 103
Harrisburg, PA 17110
Telephone: 717-234-3358
Fax: 717-234-1907
E-mail: findacure@scpscc.org
http://scpscc.org

The Sickle Cell Foundation of Georgia, Inc.
The McGhee/King Building
2391 Benjamin E. Mays
Drive S W
Atlanta, Georgia 30311
Phone: 404-755-1641
Fax: 404-755-7955
http://www.sicklecellatlaga.org/

Citizens for Quality Sickle Cell Care, Inc.
100 Arch Street
P.O. Box 702
New Britain, CT 06050
Phone: 860-223-7222
E-mail: citizens2003@yahoo.com

Sickle Cell Information Center
www.SCInfo.org

Comprehensive Sickle Cell Centers
http://www.rhofed.com/sickle/

NIH Consensus Statement: Newborn Screening for Sickle Cell Disease and other hemoglobinopathies
http://consensus.nih.gov/cons/061/
061_intro.htm

National Newborn Screening and Genetics Resource Center
http://genes-r-us.uthscsa.edu/

National Institutes of Health
Health Information—Sickle Cell
http://www.nih.gov/

The Management of Sickle Cell Disease, Final Version, July 12, 2002
http://www.nhlbi.nih.gov/
health/prof/blood/sickle/index.htm

community based sickle cell education and advocacy organization, also received funding to coordinate and provide technical assistance to the community-based programs and to disseminate best practice information nationally.

Through the years, HRSA has also funded programs in the areas of: couples counseling, psychosocial support for individuals who have sickle cell disease and their families, young adults who have sickle cell disease, transition from pediatric to adult health care services and integration into managed care health plans.

Early in 2003 during the first session of the 108th Congress, U.S. Senators James Talent (R-MO) and Charles Schumer (D-NY), along with U.S. Representatives Danny K. Davis (D-FL) and Richard Burr (R-NC), introduced the Sickle Cell Treatment Act of 2003 (S874 & HR1736). On October 22, 2004 President George W. Bush signed the American Jobs Creation Act (H.R. 4520), which contained the sickle cell amendment (Section 712, P.L. 108-357). This law amended Title XIX of the Social Security Act to include primary and secondary preventative medical strategies for children and adults who have sickle cell disease as medical assistance under the Medicaid program, and for other purposes. Specifically the law that received bipartisan, bicameral support provides for the following:

- **Increase Access to Affordable, Quality Health Care**. Funding for sickle cell disease-related services will be provided making it easier for doctors to treat individuals who have sickle cell disease by increasing the availability of physician and laboratory services that are not currently reimbursed or underreimbursed by Medicaid.

- **Enhance Services Available to Individuals Who Have Sickle Cell Disease**. States would receive a federal 50–50 funding match for nonmedical expenses related to sickle cell disease treatment such as genetic counseling, community outreach, education, and other services.

- **Create forty Sickle Cell Treatment Centers**. $10 million would be provided annually for five years for the creation of 40 Treatment Centers that will provide medical treatment, education, and other services for individuals who have sickle cell disease.

- **Establish a Sickle Cell Research Headquarters**. A National Coordinating Center, operated by the US Department of Health and Human Services (DHHS) would be created to oversee the sickle cell disease funding and the research conducted at hospitals, universities and community-based organizations in a coordinated effort to educate individuals affected by sickle cell disease and to help find a cure for the disease.

The Sickle Cell Disease Association of America, the National Medical Association, the National Association of Children's Hospitals, the National Association of Community Health Centers, the Healthcare Leadership Council, and the American Society of Hematology all endorsed the Sickle Cell Disease Act. (Schumer, 2003). Although the Sickle Cell Treatment Act was passed in 2004, only $200,000 was appropriated to establish a demonstration program and a National Coordinating Center. Senator Jim Talent (R-MO), Senator Charles Schumer (D-NY), and Senator Richard Burr (R-NC) are currently seeking support to include at least $10 million in the Fiscal Year 2006 Labor, HHS and Education Appropriations bill for grants to create the forty treatment centers to provide medical treatment, education and other services for individuals who have sickle cell disease as included in P.L. 108-357. The fight continues!

LIVING WITH SICKLE CELL DISEASE

Ginger Davis, (personal communication, January 15, 2004) a woman who has sickle cell disease summed it up very well, "Sickle cell disease is not a death sentence.... It's not a terminal disease, it's a chronic one!" Many women who have sickle disease or who are raising children who have sickle cell disease agree that it is important to learn as much as you can about the disease. Sickle cell disease is a variable disease, knowing the various complications that can occur as well as what triggers these complications can aid in minimizing and even reducing the onset of sickle cell episodes. A proper, nutritious diet, exercise, adequate hydration, and stress management all contribute to a reduction of the impact of sickle cell disease. As women, we need to be sure that we educate our children and ourselves about sickle cell disease and trait and the potential impact it may have on our lives.

Another key to living with sickle cell disease is having a good and solid support system. A support system that consists of family, friends, a medical team specially trained in sickle cell disease, and other people who live with the disease are key to living a long productive life. A good support system can help individuals who have a sickle cell disease ensure they have a sense of purpose— a sense of fulfillment, as they will know that there are others that are willing and able to help them get through. Supports can help one move from living in the "expecting pain syndrome" to the realization that although sickle cell disease is a chronic disease, it is only a small part of your life.

ADVOCACY

What can African American women do to affect a positive change as it relates to sickle cell disease? Plenty. One of the most important activities in the "fight for a cure" movement that needs to happen for sickle cell disease is to spread the word! Many people believe that sickle cell disease has "been cured" or "went away" because they haven't heard anything about it. Remember, in the United States, 1 in 12 African Americans has sickle cell trait and 1 in 400 babies are born each year with sickle cell disease, and in West and Central Africa as many as 25 percent of the population has sickle cell trait and 1–2 percent of the babies are born with a sickle cell disease. The late Alma John, a renowned community activist from New York used to say, "Each One Reach One. Each One Teach One." To energize the movement to find a cure for sickle cell disease, African American women (and others) will need to reach one and teach one.

We can start with ourselves. If we are of childbearing age, we can find out what our own hemoglobin type is in order to know the implications for our own future. We can encourage others in our community to be tested as well. We should become educated consumers. Sisters who have sickle cell disease or are raising a child who has sickle cell disease put it this way (personal communications, January 15, 2004), "We have to advocate for self—don't wait for someone else. No one will do for you what you won't do for yourself. Be your own advocate!" To increase awareness, advocates were successful in September 2004 (National Sickle Cell Awareness Month) in getting a Sickle Cell Awareness postage stamp issued through the U.S. Postal Service. We must request, purchase, and use the stamp to help increase awareness of and support for sickle cell disease.

We need to spread the word about state newborn-screening programs. Our communities should proactively request results of their baby's newborn screening results from their baby's doctor. In states where testing for sickle cell disease is not included in the newborn screening tests for every baby—we need to contact the elected officials in those states along with the Health Commissioner and Director of the State Newborn Screening Program requesting the test be added—and mobilize others to do the same.

African American women (and others) should advocate for enhancements in state newborn screening programs. Specifically, while most states' newborn-screening laws test for sickle cell disease, the testing method used to determine disease also identifies infants who have sickle cell or other hemoglobin traits. While there is no apparent benefit to the infant in knowing its carrier status at birth, it can be a benefit to the parents. If a baby is born with sickle cell or another hemoglobin trait, we know that at least one of his/her parents also has the same trait. If parents were unaware of their sickle cell status prior to the birth of the baby, they can be tested and counseled about their risks for a subsequent child having sickle cell disease.

Most agree that newborn screening test results should be available to parents of infants tested. The Council of Regional Networks for Genetic Services (CORN) has developed Guidelines for follow-up of Carriers of Hemoglobin Variants detected by Newborn Screening, which need to be considered when implementing a newborn-screening follow-up program for sickle cell disease and related hemoglobin variants.

1. Ideally, education about newborn screening, which usually includes testing sickle cell disease, should be provided to families during prenatal care—well in advance of the time of delivery.
2. A mechanism should be in place in State Newborn Screening Programs so that all results of sickle cell newborn screening can be made available to the parents of all infants who are tested.
3. Parents of all infants who are detected to be carriers of hemoglobin variants should be offered appropriate education, counseling, and testing.
4. Individuals who counsel should have appropriate training and credentialing in order to insure the highest quality or services for families of carriers detected by newborn screening.
5. Newborn screening programs should have a mechanism for monitoring and assessing the approaches to, responses to, and costs of providing carrier education and counseling service.

Supporting CORN's guidelines, advocacy can begin at the local and state level—encouraging local and state department's of health to incorporate newborn screening follow-up and sickle cell education into their infant mortality reduction initiatives. These programs target pregnant and post-partum women, offering a range of services that generally include enhanced medical visits, home visitation, outreach workers, and other supportive services. Public health programs such as Healthy Start and Title V Maternal and Child Health (MCH) programs, such as New York State's Community Health Worker Program, Perinatal Networks, Case Management, and Home Visiting Programs should be urged to provide information to the community about sickle cell disease and their state's newborn screening program; refer clients to genetic and/or sickle cell counseling; and encourage new mothers to seek out their infant's newborn screening result.

Similar programs such as Healthy Families America, Early Intervention Programs and the Women, Infants and Children feeding program (WIC) all target pregnant and postpartum women as well as women of childbearing age. These programs can readily incorporate information about sickle cell disease and newborn screening into their programs with little or no impact to their overall budgets.

We should also develop plans to work with local and national sickle cell organizations such as: the Sickle Cell Association of America, the Sickle Cell Advisory Consortium, Inc. (SCAC) in New York, South Central Pennsylvania Sickle Cell Council, the Sickle Cell Foundation of Georgia, Inc., and Citizens for Quality Sickle Cell Care, Inc. to implement a campaign to educate our religious and spiritual institutions, fraternities, sororities, civic organizations, child care centers, and more. The education should not only center on what sickle cell disease is, but also should encourage a more proactive approach which will allow the community to be informed and educated about the impact sickle cell disease may have on their families. These groups should become advocates fighting for a cure for sickle cell disease by working with elected officials to assure funding is available in federal, state and local budgets to support sickle cell research, clinical care and supportive services. Additionally, we should exercise the principle of Ujima—collective work and responsibility and providing financial support to our local and national sickle cell organizations to advance the work they are doing to educate and counsel the community, and conducting research for a cure.

National programs such as the March of Dimes can be encouraged to promote sickle cell disease during their campaigns that target the perinatal population, such as the Folic Acid campaign. In turn, sickle cell programs can educate the community about the benefits of folic acid. Other national bodies that can work together in the movement to find a cure for sickle cell disease, include the National Medical Society, the National Black Nurses Association, the National Association of Black Social Workers, the National Association for the Advancement of Colored People (NAACP) and the National Urban League. Working together in a coordinated, strategic manner we can make a difference.

We must also ensure that money for the Sickle Cell Treatment Act (P.L. 108-357) is allocated, appropriated, and implemented through the assigned agencies.

We must make a commitment to lobby strong and consistent enough to secure the funding necessary to improve the quality of life for individuals who have sickle cell disease and to find a cure.

Lenette J. Benjamin, M.D., said it well in her 2001 Year End Report as Chief Medical Officer for the Sickle Cell Disease Association of America:

We must focus on this disease on a continuum; from newborn screening to education and counseling; from and emphasis on crisis management to a focus on health maintenance, disease prevention and early intervention; and from programs that are heavily weighted towards pediatrics to programs that provide equal opportunity for infancy through adulthood. It is necessary to involve others at the medical, social and political levels. Through our interdependence we must speak with one voice and act with a common agenda in order that our purpose will gain momentum and escalate. Medicine, Science and Community: Working Together for a Cure! (Benjamin, 2001, p. 392)

REFERENCES

American Academy of Pediatrics. Newborn Screening Task Force. 2000. Newborn Screening: A blueprint for the future—A call for a national agenda on state newborn screening programs. *Pediatrics* 106:383–422.

Benjamin, L. 2001. *CMO Report*. Accessed March 5, 2005, from www.sicklecelldisease .org/cmo_rpt.htm.

Bridges, K. R. 2002. *A Brief History of Sickle Cell Disease: Sickle Cell Disease in African Tradition*. Accessed November 4, 2005, from http://sickle.bwh.harvard.edu/scd_ history.html.

CBS News. February 28, 2001. *Sickle Cell Anemia: A Forgotten Disease?* Accessed November 4, 2005, from http://cbsnews.cbs.com/stories/2002/01/31/health/prin table326932.shtml.

Gaston, M. H., J. I. Verter, G. Woods, C. Pegelowm, J. Kelleher, G. Presbury, et al. (1986). Prophylaxis with oral penicillin in children with sickle cell anemia: A randomized trial. *New England Journal of Medicine* 314:1593–99.

Health Resources and Services Administration. November 13, 2002. Grant Awards Press Release. Accessed November 4, 2005, from http://newsroom.hrsa.gov/releases/ 2002realeases/sicklecell.htm.

———. October 3, 2003. Grant Awards Press Release. Accessed November 4, 2005, from http://newsroom.hrsa.gov/releases/2003/sicklecell.htm.

———. June 15, 2005. Grant Awards Press Release. Accessed November 5, 2005, from http://www.hhs.gov/news/press/2005pres/20050615a.html.

Mayfield, E. February 1999. *New Hope for People with Sickle Cell Anemia*. Accessed November 4, 2005, from http://www.fda.gov/fdac/features/496_sick.html.

National Institutes of Health. March 19, 2003. *NIH Disease Funding Table: Special Areas of Interest*. Accessed December 7, 2003, from http://www.nih.gov/news/funding researchareas.htm.

———. September 21, 2005. *NIH Disease Funding Table: Special Areas of Interest*. Accessed November 4, 2005, from http://www.nih.gov/news/fundingresearchareas .htm.

National Institutes of Health, Consensus Conference. 1987. Newborn screening for sickle cell disease and other hemoglobinopathies. *Journal of the American Medical Association* 258:1205–9.

National Institutes of Health, National Heart, Lung and Blood Institute, Division of Blood Diseases and Resources. June, 2002a. *The Management of Sickle Cell Disease*, 4th ed. Publication No. 02-2117.

———. September, 2002b. *Sickle Cell Research for Treatment and Cure.* Publication No. 02-5214.

New York State Department of Health. Sickle Cell Advisory Committee. 2002. *Guidelines for the Treatment of People with Sickle Cell Disease*.

Novartis. 2005. Exjade® Media Release. Accessed November 4, 2005, from http://hugin .info/134323/R/1019429/160306.pdf.

Quinn, C. T., Z. R. Rogers, and G. R. Buchanan. 2004. Survival of children with sickle cell disease. *Blood* 103(11):4023–27.

Sickle Cell Disease Association of America [SCDAA], Inc. (n.d.). *Who Is Affected?* Excerpted from *A Comprehensive Guide to Sickle Cell Disease and SCDAA Services*. Accessed November 4, 2005, from http://www.sicklecelldisease.org/about_scd/affected1.phtml.

———. 2005. SCDAA responds favorably to positive review of Exjade by FDA advisory committees. Accessed November 4, 2005, from http://www.sicklecelldisease.org/news/2005/exjade_review.phtml.

South Central Pennsylvania Sickle Cell Council. n.d. *The History of Sickle Cell Disease.* Accessed November 4, 2005, from http://www.scpscc.ort/resources/history.html.

U.S. General Accounting Office. March 2003, *Newborn Screening Programs Report*, GAO-03-449.

U.S. Senator Charles Schumer. October 7, 2004. Press Release. Accessed November 4, 2005, http://schumer.senate.gov/SchumerWebsite/pressroom/press_releases/2004/PR03000.SickelCell100704.html.

5

Diabetes and African American Women

CATHERINE FISHER COLLINS

Diabetes is a silent but deadly disease, affecting an estimated 18.2 million Americans (U.S. Centers for Disease Control and Prevention [CDC], 2005). According to the Centers for Disease Control and Prevention, "diabetes is a disease in which blood glucose levels are above normal.... The pancreas, an organ that lies near the stomach, makes a hormone called insulin to help glucose get into the cells of our bodies. When you have diabetes, your body either doesn't make enough insulin or can't use its own insulin as well as it should. This causes sugar to build up in your blood" (CDC, 2005).

Between 1980 and 2003, the number of Americans diagnosed with diabetes more than doubled, growing from 5.8 million to a whopping 14.7 million (CDC, 2006). The prevalence of diabetes among African Americans is about 70 percent higher than among whites (BlackHealthCare.com, 2005). Researchers estimate that an additional 5.2 million have diabetes but have yet to be diagnosed. In addition, diabetes can "cause serious health complications including heart disease, blindness, kidney failure, and lower-extremity amputations" (CDC, 2005, p. 1).

Indeed, diabetes is the sixth-leading cause of death in the United States, contributing to 213,062 deaths in 2000 alone (CDC, 2005). However, it must be noted that diabetes is likely to be underreported as a cause of death, as "studies have found that only about 35% to 40% of decedents with diabetes have diabetes listed anywhere on the death certificate and only about 10% to 15% have it listed as the underlying cause of death" (CDC, 2005, p. 1).

This chapter is dedicated to the memory of Nellie Arzelia Thornton, July 1945–November 1995, who loved children and served as the Fourteenth National President of Jack & Jill of America, and who was my friend.

Figure 5.1
Age-Specific Prevalence of Women Diagnosed with Diabetes per 100 Population by Race, United States, 2002

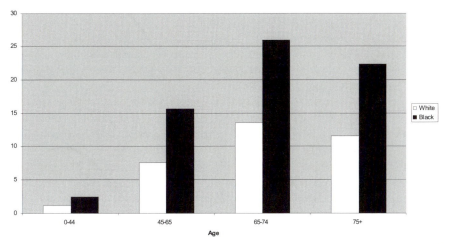

Source: U.S. Centers for Disease Control, online at cdc.gov/diabetes/statistics/prev/national/ table2002.htm, p. 1.

Diabetes is the fourth leading cause of death among African American women (Leigh & Jimenez, 2003, table p. 59); one in four black women over 55 years of age has diabetes (American Diabetes Association, 2005). This disease is a severe problem among African American women. As shown in Figure 5.1, the prevalence of diabetes among African American women in 2002 was extremely high. Even though there has been some improvement, their vulnerability to this disease is far greater than that of white women. Further, regardless of race or ethnicity, prevalence tends to be highest among persons aged 65–74 and lowest among women younger than 45 years of age.

There are two kinds of diabetes: type 1 and type 2. Type 1 diabetes, previously known as juvenile diabetes, is typically diagnosed in children and young adults. In type 1 diabetes, the body does not produce enough insulin, a substance the body needs in order to covert sugar into the fuel needed by the cells of the body.

As "ninety-five percent of African Americans with diabetes have diabetes II" (*American Legacy*, 2004, p. 92), diabetes type 2 will be the subject of this chapter. Diabetes type 2 is associated with onset in the mature adult years. Furthermore, diabetes type 2 and its effect on the body—the inability of the pancreas to produce enough insulin to regulate the amount of sugar in the blood stream—require the patient to control the diabetes by regulating the intake of food through dietary management and, if necessary, medication.

One of the strong risk factors for acquiring diabetes type 2 is obesity. In that regard, African American women are losing yet another health battle, "according to the American Obesity Association, 78 percent of African American women are overweight [and] 51 percent [are] obese" (Kinnon, 2004, p. 93). And "some recent evidence show that the degree to which obesity is a risk factor for diabetes may depend on the location of excess weight. Truncal, or upper body obesity, is a great risk factor for type 2 diabetes, compared to excess weight carried below the waist . . . and [the] study showed that African Americans have a greater tendency to develop upper body obesity, which increases their risk to type 2 diabetes (BlackHealthCare.com, 2005).

Diabetes is even more dangerous because it is a precursor for heart disease, strokes, colon cancer, gallbladder disease, endometrial cancer, lower-leg amputation, osteoarthritis, complications of pregnancy, poor female reproductive health, and sleep apnea (Kinnon, 2004, p. 93).

According to the American Diabetes Association (2005, p.1), "heart disease strikes people with diabetes more than twice as often as it strikes people without diabetes. People with diabetes are five times more likely to suffer strokes and once having had a stroke, are two to four times as likely to have a recurrence. Deaths from heart disease in women with diabetes have increased 23% over the past 30 years compared to a 27% decrease in women without diabetes." Further, "diabetes is the most frequent cause of non-traumatic lower limb amputations. The risk of a leg amputation is 15 to 40 times greater for a person with diabetes. More than 60% of nontraumatic lower-limb amputations in the U.S. occur among people with diabetes. Each year, 82,000 people lose their foot or leg to diabetes. Among people with diabetes, African Americans are 1.5 to 2.5 times more likely to suffer from lower limb amputations" (American Diabetes Association, 2005).

Also disturbing is the apparent connection between diabetes and the risk of developing Alzheimer's disease, which affects the brain and memory of 4 million people in the United States (Petit & Adamec, 2002, p. 21; "Long term study," 2004). Further, according to Petit and Adamec (2002), "people with diabetes are three times more likely to suffer from depression than nondiabetics . . . [and] women with diabetes are more likely to be diagnosed with depression than men" (p. 75).

Because of diabetes-related health complications, African American women with diabetes must keep current on all medical treatment/management options that may have positive or adverse effects on their health status, as evidenced in the case of a diabetic named Alley (Shute, 2004).

Alley decided to seek cosmetic surgery. It was reported that "when Alley, then 47 talked to the surgeon John Pinnella, about liposuction in November 2000, she [said that] 'he assured me it was 100 percent fantastic for diabetics' " (Shute, 2004, p. 58). Alley paid $2,700 and had the surgery. One day after surgery, she was too ill to make her first follow-up visit. It was reported that, two weeks later, she was hospitalized with a massive infection. Alley, "suffered blood clots, required a colostomy . . . [and] after nine months of repeated infections and hospitalizations, both legs above the knees were amputated. [Now] Alley's at home sitting in a wheelchair" (p. 58).

Despite such horror stories, modern medicine has advanced in the past decade and has incorporated new home blood glucose monitors, human insulin, new medicines, insulin pumps, and the transplants of islet cells and the pancreas. All of these advances have had a positive impact on diabetes management.

Nonetheless, diabetes still requires careful management through continuous stress reduction management and monitoring of lifestyle behavior. Also, African American women must stay current on all medical and social information regarding their health, especially when they have chronic illnesses.

IMPACT OF THE HISTORICAL TREATMENT OF AFRICAN AMERICAN WOMEN AND WHY SOME FAIL TO SEEK NEEDED MEDICAL TREATMENT

In order to control lifestyle and inappropriate health behavior/practices, African American women must have access to understandable health information from competent health care providers. African American women, who are knowledgeable about the historical mistreatment of their ancestors, are often reluctant to trust the health system. Some have gained access to competent health care providers. However, "they are reminded that even with health access, their ancestors were subjected to discrimination and horrific medical abuses, such as injection with tuberculosis and syphilis bacteria, and impromptu limb amputation by white physicians eager to show medical students the latest surgical techniques" (Johnson, 1994, p. 54).

In one such case—as shown in the theater and television productions of "Miss Evers' Boys," which depicted the 1932 "Tuskegee Study of Untreated Syphilis in the Negro Male"—the federal government funded a long-term study of syphilis, seeking to learn how syphilis affected Blacks, as opposed to whites. The study withheld treatment from the 400 poor, Black men involved in the study, who were told only that they were being treated for "bad blood." Forty years later, a newspaper exposed the experiment to the public, and the government ended the study. By the end of the experiment, 28 of the men had died directly of syphilis, 100 were dead of related complications, 40 of their wives had been infected, and 19 of their children had been born with congenital syphilis (Brunner, 2005).

The media also helps to further educate the American public regarding the atrocities committed by the medical profession. Another example of this is the widely televised case of the African American whose unaffected leg was mistakenly amputated by a Florida physician.

Further, Beardsley (1990) provided an excellent historical account of health care provided to African American women between 1900 and 1930, a period he calls the "Era of Denial." In Beardsley's historical account, he discusses how African American women were denied access to health professionals and hospital services. This accounted for numerous childbirth deaths of both mothers and infants, as well as raging tuberculosis and syphilis. Also noted by Beardsley was the "scourge of American black women," other causes of high morbidity, diabetes among them. This historical account and others has helped create a sense of mistrust and apprehension among African American women who are diabetics about seeking medical attention.

While there is a scarcity of data prior to 1940, current data suggest that diabetes was a serious illness then, especially for women over fifty (Beardsley,

1990). There is, however statistics from surveys carried out in the early 1920s that note the rise in the rates of diabetes type 2 in Blacks, particularly Black women, as well as a higher rate of diabetes mortality and complications in the Black community. As Beardsley points out, cardiovascular and renal disease were then, as they are now, severe complications of diabetes and were, by 1900, among the greatest killers of Blacks (p. 128).

In 1900, African American women had the highest mortality rate—a fact that, over 100 years later, is still true, according to U.S. governmental agencies. Following the end of World War I, limited gains in health conditions were experienced by African American women. The Great Depression served as the force that essentially eliminated some of the public health clinics/programs (Collins, 1996, p. 3). The Depression also took a heavy toll on African Americans, who were forced out of jobs to make room for unemployed whites (Beardsley, 1990), thus eliminating their ability to pay for health care. It was not until the passage of the 1935 Social Security Act that some clinics in poor neighborhoods were reestablished.

As Beardsley (1990) points out, the access of African American women to health services increased after the federal government's Hill-Burton Act of 1946, which provided resources to build hospitals. With federal intervention, some hospitals admitted African American women to segregated hospital wards, many of which were understaffed, poorly equipped, and attended by racist white physicians. Even though African American women were able to use hospital services in their community, there were no guarantees that they would receive quality care. Hospital policies impacted their care, where "expectant black mothers were particularly victimized by Chicago racism: their own black hospitals often had no space for them, yet many maternity beds lay empty in white hospitals" (p. 137).

A well-devised and defined segregated health care delivery system had developed, with one tier for Blacks and one for whites. This segregated health care system would ultimately be challenged by the National Association for the Advancement of Colored People (NAACP), and the overt discrimination in health care became less distinguishable, because of potential loss of federal funding and the ability to sue under the Civil Rights Act of 1964.

By the 1970s, which Beardsley calls the "Era of Attempted Restitution," the civil rights movement had opened some doors to health care. However, racism and its effects could still be found in hospitals built with federal dollars. In certain southern hospitals, African American women were hospitalized in segregated wards that often lacked equipment that was available in the white wards/wings of the same hospital. The Hill Burton federal program, coupled with other federal initiatives (Social Security) failed to arrest the incredible mortality rate of this era, where the death rate of Black women was 60 percent above that of white women, and the rate of Black men was 45 percent above their white counterparts (Beardsley, p. 138). Even with the programs previously mentioned and the new programs of the 1990s, African American women have remained in poor health.

From the historical data presented here, it is evident that diabetes has and continue to have a disproportionate affect on African American women. It exists as a fact, leaving no need for debate. What does need to be addressed, is how we can impact on this plague.

All too often we look at socioeconomic status, poverty, access to health care, and level of education as the culprits in answering questions regarding the poor health status of African American women. This is not to say that those factors are not contributors to ill health. However, it should also be noted that there are "45 million Americans who are uninsured, which is 15.6% of the population" (Appleby, 2004, p. 48). The fact that that uninsured segment of the population includes a large number of African Americans, when coupled with racism, severely compromises the health status of African American women. Indeed, racism and the stress precipitated by it are etiologic factors in diabetes type 2 and the health complications that result from diabetes—complications that must be considered in diseases that have such a deplorable outcome.

Racism and racists who create stressful situations for African American women can manipulate the environment in such a fashion that the resulting stress can affect the diabetic's physical well-being. Clearly, research has proven that stress will increase blood pressure (Newberry et al., 1991), heart rate (Derrick, 1997), genital herpes recurrences (Schmidt et al., 1985), and decreased renal excretion of salt, resulting in increased fluid retention (Newberry et al., 1991). In addition, stress has been shown to have a detrimental impact on an individual's immune system (Collins, 2003), thus lowering resistance to infection—a complication of diabetes which often results in "black patients undergoing twice as many amputations as whites" (U.S. Department of Health and Human Services, 1992).

There are many research studies in which it is reported that stress has a negative impact on the immune system. For example, dental students' antibody levels were found to be significantly lowered before final examinations (Jemmott & Locke, 1984). Also, there is evidence that unemployed women had a reduction in white blood cells when compared to employed women (Arnetz et al., 1987).

Additional studies, by Kiecolt-Glaser and Glaser (1987), reported changes in immune systems of medical students during examinations. The researchers also and noted the impact of stress on the immune systems of recently separated women, when compared to those of married women. There is no doubt that immunosupression can be caused or exacerbated by stress. How far the stress of racism extends in depressing the function of the immune system function requires a much more in-depth approach—too lengthy for this chapter. However, Collins (2003) shows how the impact of racism in a variety of settings including work and home adversely affect the health status of African American women. We must, therefore, control stressful situations arising out of racism.

Is this possible? According to (Johnson, 1994), most African Americans will be treated by white physicians—only 3 percent of U.S. physicians are Black— "whose training and culture interfere with their good judgment. In short, their actions are racially motivated" (Johnson, 1994, p. 55). Johnson continues to explain how "racism rears its ugly head in the doctor's offices" (p. 55), presenting an analysis of a study by Dr. David Levy, a Houston family practitioner who investigated five ways race affects the doctor/patient relationship. As

I present them, imagine that you are an overweight African American female patient with diabetes type 2.

According to Dr. Levy, racism raises its ugly head when a white physician shows their disrespect for a Black patient by attending to a white patient who arrives after them, or begins an examinatin without introducing himself. On the other side of the problem is the white physician who overidentifies with a Black patient, giving advice on how she should live her life, or is ignorant of the importance of considering how African American culture impacts on behavior.

White physicians, who proclaim to be "colorblind" in their care giving, are also a detriment to the African American patient, because the physician fails to acknowledge the importance of race differences (e.g., health practices) which may need to be considered in the treatment plan.

Dr. Levy's fifth example is the physician who makes assumptions about all African Americans based on his experiences with a few. This physician stereotypes all African Americans, without consideration of individual differences.

SOCIAL SUPPORT AND BUFFERS OF STRESS ASSOCIATED WITH RACISM AND DIABETIC PROGRAMS

African American women who encounter the kind of racism described by Dr. Levy—or other forms of racism, whether at work, at school, while shopping— must shield themselves from the stress induced by these encounters of these individuals, whom I call psychological terrorists. To buffer one's self from racism induced by our social and health care system, African American women must turn to their social support network, which research has shown can alleviate the impact of stressful life events and their effects on health outcomes.

Some have posited that females with a strong social support system are much better prepared to cope with life stressors. Those who do not have strong social support systems can suffer dreadful results, such as poor physical and mental health. Social support can come from a variety of sources. One key supporting structure appear to be the church; another is the family.

In research conducted by Brown and Gray (1987), 451 Black adults—60 percent of who were female—were observed to ascertain the level of relationship of social support and health outcomes. Five variables were used: nearby relatives, confidants, neighbors, religiosity, and perceived social support. One of the study's findings supports the importance of religious participation. The study found that "increased frequency of participation in religious activities for black females is a way of coping with the ill health of loved ones and minimizing its effect on one's own physical health" (p. 171).

In a later study, Brown et al. (1990) found that Blacks with the least amount of religious participation had higher depressive symptoms, which seems to further validate the importance of the church. However, there have been studies with mixed results regarding the effects of religion on depression (Dressler, 1991). When exploring African Americans in church, women can and do "bring their problems to the Lord." This is done through the Black church's rituals of "shouting," "dancing," deep religious meditation, testimonials, singing, and praising God. The theology of the sermon also serves as a teacher or counselor to help place the racist world into the context of the evil, mean-spirited antics of the devil. All of these rituals serve as tension relievers and as basic survival techniques.

No other institution has aided the Black community more than the Black church, where congregations are disproportionately African American women. The church provides unlimited resources, food, shelter, counseling, and spiritual guidance (Wilmore, 1973). In the face of mounting social unrest of the 1960s, the church leadership (e.g., Dr. Martin Luther King Jr.) was the first social institution to publicly speak out against American racism. Thus the church provides a spiritual outlet for stress associated with racism.

As previously mentioned, obesity among African American women is of epidemic proportions (Kinnon, 2004), and disproportionately so among Black church congregations. Studies by Brown and Gray (1987) and Brown et al. (1990) have shown that religion/spirituality has some impact on the elevation of stress that may affect diabetic outcomes. Some Black churches have established programs designed to empower their congregations—which are typically disproportionately composed of African American women—to take control of their health. In one such initiative called "Project Power," church leaders do everything from conducting cooking classes to starting fitness ministries. In Norfolk, Virginia, members of First Baptist Church participate in bicycle races sponsored by the American Diabetes Association (Chappell, 2005).

In Los Angeles, a church project on diabetes begins with a kickoff breakfast where community leaders introduce the program's intent and concept. Health professionals from the American Diabetes Association (ADA) and the chairman of the association's Cultural Diversity Program were featured speakers, providing current evidence of the seriousness of diabetes among African Americans nationwide. Utilizing the efforts of the California Blue Cross, 200 churches were targeted for information sessions ("Black Church Diabetes Program," 1994).

Another program was initiated in upstate New York. The ADA's Cultural Diversity Program spearheaded this church congregation-directed program. A breakfast was also held with church pastors and other clergy to introduce them to the seriousness of diabetes among the community and their congregations. The diabetes program was appropriately entitled "Diabetes Sunday," and was presented to inner-city community block clubs and church congregations, who heard speakers and saw food demonstrations.

The Black church is one of several avenues that can be used to reach at-risk overweight African American women. Another is the diabetes health education programs. One such program is PATHWAYS. Program participants were thirteen overweight African American women with a minimum of three months of treatment history for diabetes type 2 and at least 120 percent of ideal body weight. The PATHWAYS program took reading levels into account to assure that the client could read educational materials, and utilized adult learning guidelines in presenting educational information. This program also gradually introduced dietary changes with a program guide that included ethnic foods (e.g., salt pork, ham hocks, greens) and a walking/exercise program. Of the ten participants who completed the eighteen-week program, a loss of 9–10 pounds was noted, and after one year, an average weight loss of 9.8 pounds was reported. As the participants lost weight, their blood sugar values improved substantially (McNabb et al., 1993).

PATHWAYS included cultural consideration and adult learning style, which may have contributed significantly to its success. The program reported that behavior modification and lifestyle behavior changes were considered in working with this population. Religiosity as a variable was not mentioned in the PATHWAYS program design. However, because African American women are in disproportionate numbers among the Black church congregations (Collins, 2003, p. 84), religiosity as a helping or reinforcement variable in health maintenance efforts (e.g., control weight gain) might be worth future investigation.

Overall, the aim of most diabetes education programs should include, at a minimum: a physical exercise component; classes in how to eat a heart-healthy diet, high in fiber that includes oat bran, oatmeal, whole grain breads; a how-to loss weight program for overweight clients; and smoking cessation and blood pressure monitoring components. No one will deny that the health status of African American women is poor, and a contributing factor is diabetes type 2 and its complications, which are associated with poor health management and health practices. Epidemiological evidence clearly indicates that obesity—which is perpetuated by a "poverty diet" high in fat and sweets and low in vegetables and fruits—and a health care industry and social structure riddled with racial discrimination and racism combine in contributing to stress, lowering bodily defenses and thus assuring poor health outcomes.

Furthermore, the impact on the health status of African American women by those who are insensitive to cultural differences, as well as the restricted level of access to the health care industry and services, will continue to increase health care costs with little or no return in healthy lifestyle. Heretofore, we have relied heavily on the health care industry to help alleviate the health ills of African American women who suffer with diabetes. Efforts in diabetes health education have been designed that meet most of the physical health needs of African American women. However, they need to be able to trust the system in order to feel comfortable in availing themselves of these services. These diabetic education programs have been designed most often within a medical or health behavioral model approach. Varying degrees of success have been noted in this chapter and in the literature.

However, health educators must also consider the impact of, and take a closer look at, utilizing the spirituality of African American women in program design. With the ever-increasing number of African American women being diagnosed with diabetes, the traditional health education approach, as well as the not-so-traditional (e.g., the church/spirituality), should be given serious consideration.

REFERENCES

American Diabetes Association. 2005. *Diabetes Statistics for African Americans*. Accessed March 6, 2006, from http://diabetes.org/diabetes-statistics/african-ameri cans.jsp. "Taking Control of Diabetes Risks." Summer 2004. *American Legacy: the Magazine of African-America Story and Culture* 10, no. 2.

Appleby, J. August 27, 2004. "Ranks of Uninsured Grow to Highest Since '98." *USA Today,* p. 48.

Arnetz B. B., J. Wasserman, B. Petrini, S. O. Brenner, L. Levi, P. Eneroth, H. Salovaara, R. Hjelm, L. Salovaara, T. Theorell, and I. Peterson. 1987. "Immune Function in Unemployed Women." *Psychosomatic Medicine* 49, 3–12.

Beardsley, E. May 1990. "Race as a Factor in Health." In Rim Apple, ed., *Women's Health and Medicine in America: A Historical Handbook.* New York: Garland.

"Black Church Diabetes Program Gets Underway in Los Angeles." September 22, 1994. *Los Angeles Sentinal,* p. A10:1.

BlackHealthCare.com. 2005. "Diabetes in African Americans."

Brown, D., and L. Gray. Winter, 1987. "Social Support and Physical and Mental Health of Urban Black Adults." *Journal of Human Stress,* 13, 165–74.

Brown, D., S. Nilubuisi, and L. Gray. 1990. "Religiosity and Psychological Distress Among Blacks." *Journal of Religion and Health,* 29, 55–68.

Brunner, B. 2005. The Tuskegee Syphilis Experiment: The U.S. Government's 40-Year Experiment on Black Men with Syphilis. Accessed July 29, 2005, from http://www.infoplease.com/spot/bhmtuskegee1.html.

Chappell, K. March 2005. "Diabetes Treatment, Research and Cure." *Ebony,* pp. 126–28.

Collins, C. F. 2003. *Sources of Stress and Relief for African-American Women.* Westport, CT: Praeger.

Collins, C. F., ed. 1996. *African American Women's Health and Social Issues.* Westport, CT: Praeger.

Derrick, R. March 1997. "Healing the Wounds of Racism." *Essence,* pp. 35–37.

Dressler, W. 1991. *Stress and Adaptation in the Context of Culture: Depression in a Southern Black Community.* Albany, NY: State University of New York at Albany.

Jemmott, J. B., III, and S. E. Locke. 1984. "Psychosocial Factors: Immunologic Mediation and Human Susceptibility to Infectious Disease: How Much Do We Know?" *Psychological Bulletin* 95, 78–108.

Johnson, K. A. Spring 1994. "The Color of Health Care." *Heart and Soul,* pp. 53–57.

Kiecolt-Glaser, J. K., and R. Glaser. 1987. "Psychosocial Moderators of Immune Functions." *Annals of Behavioral Medicine* 9(2):16–20, 140–212.

Kinnon, Joy B. July 2004 "Taking It Off." *Ebony,* pp. 93–96.

Leigh, W., and M. Jimenez. 2003. *Women of Color Health Data Book.* Washington, D.C.: National Institutes of Health, Office of The Director.

"Long-term Study Links Diabetes to Increased Risk of Alzheimer's." May 31, 2004. *Los Angeles Business Journal.*

McNabb, W. L., M. T. Quinn, and L. Rosing. 1993. "Weight Loss Program for Inner-city Black Women with Non-insulin Dependent Diabetes Mellitus." *PATHWAYS, Journal of American Diabetes Association* 93, 75–77.

Newberry, B., J. Jaikin-Modden, and T. J. Gerstenberger. 1991. *A Holistic Conceptualization of Stress and Disease.* New York: AMS Press.

Petit, W. A., and C. Adamec. 2002. *The Encyclopedia of Diabetes.* Facts on File Library of Health and Living. New York: Facts on File.

Schmidt, D. D., S. Zyanski, J. Ellnet, and M. L. Kiemer. 1985. "Stress as a Precipitating Factor in Recurrent Herpes Labialis." *Journal of Family Practice* 20, 359–366.

Shute, N. May 31, 2004. "Makeover Nation." *U.S. News and World Report,* pp. 53–63.

Stack, C. 1974. *All Our Kin: Strategies for Survival in a Black Community.* New York: Harper & Row.

U.S. Center for Disease Control. National Center for Chronic Diseases, Prevention, and Health Promotion. "Frequently Asked Questions." Accessed May 10, 2005, from http://www.cdc.gov/diabetes/FAQ/basic.htm, p. 1.

———. "Data Trends National Diabetes Surveillance System." Accessed March 6, 2006, from http://www.dcd.gov/diabetes/statistics/prev/national/figpersons.htm.

———. Publication and Products. National Diabetes Fact Sheet, National Estimates on Diabetes. Accessed May 10, 2005, from http://www.cdc.gov/diabetes/pubs/estimates.htm#deaths, p. 1.

U.S. Department of Health and Human Services. November 1992. "Diabetes in Black Americans." Fact Sheet, National Diabetes Information Clearinghouse, NO93-326.

Wilmore, G. 1973. *Black Religion and Black Radicalism.* Garden City, NY: Anchor Books.

6

HIV/AIDS: Confronting the Health Risk Factors

LORRAINE E. PEELER

Epidemic, pandemic, endemic, disproportionate, escalation, and *epicenter* are words that have been directly associated with human immunodeficiency virus/ acquired immune deficiency syndrome (HIV/AIDS) and the African American community. Unfortunately, over the past years these words have been descriptors about HIV/AIDS and African American women. These are words that we do not use on a daily basis but have serious implications as it relates to our health.

Let us put these words in context as they relate to the African American community. HIV/AIDS is epidemic because it is a deadly disease and because it has spread rapidly and extensively by infection and affects many people. It is endemic because once the epicenter shifted from the Gay community, the disease has hovered in the African American community, infecting women, children, and men. It is pandemic because now HIV/AIDS is widespread, prevalent, and common in African American communities. The impact of the epidemic is similar in African American communities in major cities and in rural communities. It is geographically widespread in this country, specifically urban and rural centers where African Americans live, which could be due to cultural beliefs that lead to similar behaviors. In 1999, more African Americans were reported with AIDS than any other racial/ethnic group, according to the most recent Center for Disease Control (CDC) figures for that year.

The disease disproportionately affects the African American community. It is unbalanced in it is impact on our community in proportion to the white community. The National Institutes of Health (2003) defines health disparities as "differences in the incidence, prevalence, mortality and burden of disease and other adverse health conditions that exist among specific population groups in the United States" (http://healthdisparities.nih.gov/faqs.html). For African

Americans in most instances, including HIV/AIDS, when we are infected, the probability of death is higher than in the majority population.

Initially, in addition, rates of infection have escalated since 1993. The epicenter has shifted from the gay community to communities of color, specifically African Americans. This means that what was the center from which the virus radiated is no longer the center. The focus of the disease has shifted to our community, and many of us are still ignorant about how the virus spreads and who is at risk.

Originally HIV/AIDS was concentrated in major cities like San Francisco, Miami, New York City, and Los Angeles, and among those termed "socially deviant" people. It appeared that other sectors of the population would be spared. This continued to foster an erroneous belief system that HIV/AIDS was not a disease that African Americans needed to concern themselves with. While African Americans were crystallizing these beliefs, HIV/AIDS became prevalent in deteriorating inner-city communities due to behaviors that we did not know led to infection, like intravenous drug use, the sex trade business, unprotected sex with these individuals, and ignorance and/or denial about male partners and spouses who had multiple partners and/or are on the "down low," sleeping with other men. These misperceptions contributed significantly to the disproportionate representation of the disease in African American communities in the United States.

Even though these descriptors are true, most African Americans, especially women, do not believe that this disease can directly infect or affect their life. *Ignorance is not bliss!* Ignorance can and does lead to death. It is time out for this reign of ignorance because African American women's health and lives are at risk, and at alarming rates. In addition, the majority of the research literature on African American women and HIV/AIDS focuses on persons who are economically disadvantaged and ages 18–44 years old. The research needs to address the full range of African American women, despite social class, age and/or education, because the whole spectrum of this population is at risk.

HIV/AIDS—A COMPLEX DISEASE

The question may come up about why is this discussion about a disease any different than talking to African American women about breast cancer, hypertension, or heart disease? It is a different and necessary matter to address the impact of HIV/AIDS in our community, because the disease is complex. But complexity describes the state of understanding African American women and health issues in general. Roberson (1996) asserts that there are three indicators needed to assess African American women and their health. The indicators are: African American women's placement in the social structure that influences health and illnesses; societal stereotypes about African American women's health-related behaviors, and the health status situation of African American women that impact disease occurrences.

McNair and Prather (2004) are more specific about African American women's health and HIV/AIDS. They summarize research on this perspective and outline the factors that influence African American women's increased risk of acquiring HIV/AIDS. Similar to Roberson, they believe the factors are related to the intersection of race, gender, and social class in the lives of African American women, which gives rise to conditions that are associated with HIV risks. They summarize the factors that are directly related to HIV risks and African American women on two dimensions: social and contextual. Social factors are variables that impact groups of people similarly but are external to the individuals, like cultural beliefs, values, and practices. Contextual factors are environmental variables that influence an individual's perspective and therefore have import only for that person, such as relationship history, victimization experience, and levels of environmental stress.

There is a definite intersection of variables that influence African American women and the potential of contracting HIV/AIDS. African American women are increasingly at risk because there is no straight line between our potential exposure and issues that complicate health-promoting behaviors. Specifically, social structure and societal stereotypes are part of the social construction of HIV/AIDS in the African American community. The complexity of this disease impacts some fundamental issues that go beyond our sexual behavior and delves into the motivators of our behaviors that ignore warning signs and caution lights as well as clear and present dangers. It deals with our myths, stereotypes, lies, and taboos related to our sexual lives, our sexuality, and our social-psychological beliefs.

HIV/AIDS is not just a disease in the African American community, it is a symbol. A symbol is something that represents something else by association, and it can represent knowledge with encrypted beliefs. Washington (2000) states that symbols guide the way in which we look at the world. Symbols convey the knowledge, wisdom, myths, and traditions of a people. The history of the societal response to HIV/AIDS has had an effect on African American views about this disease. The initial reports regarding HIV/AIDS describe and allude to a perception of the disease as impacting persons who are socially deviant and support a certain lifestyle, which includes white homosexual and bisexual men (DiClemente, 1992; Kimberly & Serovich, 1999). Furthermore, infected individuals and the areas where they resided were held in very low esteem. Consequently, African Americans began to associate the disease with negative symbols.

By the time HIV/AIDS became a household word in the African American community, it was associated with a "deviant" lifestyle. Homosexual (gay) men were the transmitters and the recipients of the virus. It was not a disease that "good black girls" had to concern themselves with—unless they had a son who was in that lifestyle. Even our male preachers helped us to process this growing epidemic, not as a disease but a social/moral issue. Pittman et al. (1992) assert that misperceptions of risk for HIV among African American women appear to have resulted partly from early emphasis of AIDS as a disease of white, gay males. The African American preachers told us that HIV/AIDS was God's curse on this deviant lifestyle (even if it was our sons, brothers, or nephew who contracted it). The African American pastor's perspective was that HIV/AIDS was "God's curse on homosexuals." So we, African American women, believed this was an issue (not a disease), which disease was not our problem. It was the problem of the "other" people. Unfortunately the processing of this communicable disease as a social/moral issue has promoted ignorance and death for many African American women.

This platform of ignorance has laid the groundwork for where we are today as it relates to this disease. It is important to note that HIV/AIDS is not only a sexually transmitted disease, it is a socially transmitted disease and contraction has psychological implications. HIV/AIDS is at epidemic proportions in our community, and African American women contract the virus at higher rates than any other group in this country. Somewhere, someone did not talk plainly to us about this disease, and we got lulled asleep by the song of ignorance and complacency.

DEMOGRAPHICS

There are many speculations and conjectures about why there has been the dramatic shift of the epicenter of HIV/AIDS epidemic. Haverkos and Turner (1999) suggest that these differences might be due to factors like socioeconomic issues that affect access to treatment, drug abuse, and sexual behavior. Some believe that the rise of the HIV/AIDS epidemic in communities of color comes, not just from one factor, but from many factors. Some of the factors include: poor health due to social and economic inequities; failure to access and trust community and health institutions due to sociocultural reasons like race, ethnicity, and being multiple minorities due to membership in subpopulations like substance users; and gay/bisexual men who have sex with men, women, youth, and prison inmates. Additional factors are lack of education about the reality of the disease, perpetuation of myths and stereotypes about the disease, and denial about risky behaviors (New York State AIDS Advisory Council, 2000/2001).

General

Over ten years ago, the rise in HIV/AIDS cases for African Americans began to be tracked and the ominous prediction was that the incidence in the African American community was going to escalate. According to DiClemente (1992), African American men and women were 10 times more likely to acquire AIDS from a heterosexual relationship rather than a same-sex relationship. Wingood and DiClemente (1998) suggested that the wealth of demographic data indicated that the HIV epidemic will continue to exact a disproportionately higher toll among African American women unless programs are developed that promote the adoption and maintenance of HIV prevention practices.

Haverkos and Turner (1999) state that AIDS among African Americans and Hispanics is reported to occur at a significantly higher rate than among whites. In 1999, more African Americans were reported with AIDS than any other racial or ethnic group, according to the most recent Centers for Disease Control (CDC) figures, confirming the prediction of the shift to the African American community and the impending escalation. These statistics were staggering because African Americans represent only an estimated 12 percent of the total U.S. population, but make up almost 37 percent of all AIDS cases reported in this country and nearly half (47 percent) of all new infections recorded in 1999, a rate more than twice that for Hispanics and eight times greater than the rate for whites.

Williams et al. (2003) asserted that current research estimated that between 240,000 and 325,000 African Americans are infected by HIV. This situation has resulted in 10 to 15 times the risk of HIV infections among African American females compared to their white counterparts. Not only is the contraction rate for African American females astronomical, but the mortality rate for African American women, as compared to white women, is much higher than the national average.

Women Specific

The impact of HIV/AIDS in the African American community has soared, especially for African American women. Demographic information from 1993 until 2003 supports the importance of the shift and impact. All statistical data indicate that African American women are disproportionately represented among AIDS cases (Wingood & DiClemente, 1998; CDC, 2002). Fifty-four percent of the AIDS cases reported are African American women. African American women accounted for approximately 64 percent of HIV cases reported among women, overall. Specifically, the rate of infection among African American women ages 20–44 is astronomical. From 1994 to 1998, approximately 80 per 100,000 women African American were infected, a number four times higher than Latinas of the same age and sixteen times higher than the rates of white women (CDC, 2003). Seniors are not exempt from the epidemic because 70 percent of the women over 50 with AIDS are African American and Hispanic (HIV/AIDS, 2004). In addition, studies indicate that there is a direct link between sexually transmitted diseases (STDs) and increased risk of HIV transmission.

HIV/AIDS is the leading cause of death for African American women ages 25–34, and the disease is among the top three leading causes of death for African American women ages 35–44. Researchers estimate that 240,000–325,000 African Americans (about 1 in 50 African American men and 1 in 160 African American women) are now infected with HIV. Between 1993 and 2001, the proportion of African Americans' AIDS cases accounted for by women increased by 40 percent (CDC, 2002). As of December 2001, approximately 82,000 AIDS cases had been reported among African American women accounting for 58 percent of cumulative cases among adolescent and adult women of every racial and ethnic group (CDC, 2002). The AIDS incidence rate for African American women is 47.8 per 100,000. This is approximately 5 times the rate of the U.S. population and represents almost two-thirds of all cases diagnosed among women (CDC, 2002).

These statistics are alarming, especially when the majority of the African American population still associates HIV/AIDS with a gay lifestyle and not a heterosexual lifestyle. These specific demographics have an impact on the growth of HIV/AIDS in our community—especially among African American women and the choices that they make regarding their sexual behaviors.

FACTORS THAT MAKE US AT RISK

It easier to identify physical factors that may be responsible for the increase of HIV/AIDS transmission to African American women, but we must understand that HIV is a social disease and address that the psychosocial factors that have impacted the epidemic for African American women. This understanding is crucial because it is these factors that have left us most vulnerable to the epidemic.

There are many theories about why and how HIV is transmitted in the African American community. These perspectives range from individual, community and social issues, to social cognitive variables, health belief models, and theories of gender and power. More recently, researchers have focused more on the social context, which includes historical, social, situational, health, and chemical substances.

The literature supports the hypothesis that social factors are the predominant variables in the high rate of contraction of HIV/AIDS among African American women. McNair and Prather (2004) identify four social factors that are unique to the HIV/AIDS epidemic as it relates to African American women. The uniqueness of these factors is that the exposure for the women is through heterosexual contact. These social factors are: (1) the sex-ratio imbalance, (2) low levels of condom use, (3) multiple partners, and (4) bisexuality among African American men. I include a fifth factor, low levels of health literacy, because there is a direct correlation between health literacy and health-promoting behaviors. Let us look at each one of these areas specifically.

The Sex-Ratio Imbalance

Marital status (married, single, divorced) has influenced the epidemic of HIV/ AIDS in the African American community. Jones and Shorter-Gooden (2003) speak to the issue of sex-ratio imbalance and assert that the rate of marriage among African Americans is declining. Specifically, the 2000 U.S. Census identified 38 percent of African American women ages 18 and older as having never married. In contrast, 18 percent of white women and 25 percent of Hispanic women in this age group had never married. Moreover, the divorce rate for African American women is higher than all other women in this country.

The sex-ratio imbalance theory is summarized as the fact that women may perceive and behave with less power in their relationships and give men more disproportionate power when there is an overabundance of women in certain communities (Guttentag & Secord, 1983). Hearn and Jackson (2002) assert that African American women's behavior in intimate relationships is correlated with the ratio of men to women in the community. Specifically, in most communities there are more African American women than men.

Jones and Shorter-Gooden (2003) assert that racial oppression and the lack of economic opportunities are two of the culprits of the sex-ratio imbalance. There are also high rates of homicide, suicide, and imprisonment among African American men. Black women outnumber Black men by roughly 19 women to 17 men. There are some other culprits as well. African Americans tend to adopt popular culture quickly and without assessing long-term results. Things like shacking-up, living together, single parenthood as a lifestyle, and sharing a man have became the buzzwords and acceptable standards in our communities. On the other hand, white America has shifted away from the sexual freedom of the 1960s and 1970s, while teen parenting and single parenting continued to increase for Black communities throughout the 1980s and early 1990s.

Low Levels of Condom Use

For African American women, low levels of condom use represents a complex issue.

The fact that African American women contract HIV/AIDS at an alarming rate is evidence that "safe sex" is not a priority. Various studies (Wingood & DiClemente, 1998; McNair & Prather, 2004) report a high rate of not using condoms use among African American women for a variety of reasons that include: perceived inconvenience of using condoms as impeding spontaneity; perceived negative impact of using condoms on sexual enjoyment, especially as reported by their male partner; and the belief that using condoms negatively impacts relationship trust. Participants in these studies report that if they ask their partner to use a condom, there is an unpleasant implication that the partner is engaging in sexual activity with others.

If the rate of contraction of HIV/AIDS is the highest in the country for African American women, then we must make a direct correlation that a significant portion of these women consistently engage in unprotected sex. If they are continuing to engage in unprotected sex based on perceptions and beliefs, then we need to understand and address the power of perceptions and beliefs. Interventions need to be made on the perceptions and beliefs level.

African American women's responses to their partner's reaction to condom use is life threatening. A study by Overby and Kegeles (1994) of African American women ages 13 to 19 found that 26 percent felt they had little control over whether a condom is used during intercourse. Moreover, 75 percent agreed that if a male partner knows that the woman is taking oral contraceptives, the male does not want to use a condom. A majority of this sample believed that a male sex partner would be hurt, insulted, angry, or suspicious if questioned about his HIV risk factors. In addition, other studies of African American women found that there is a direct correlation between relationship violence and adverse sexual health behaviors (Wingood & DiClemente, 1997; Wingood et al., 2001). Overall, women usually take responsibility for contraception but often do not insist on using contraception if they fear abuse (Wyatt et al., 1998). This abuse could be physical or emotional, especially if men display anger when asked to use a condom.

The issue is that condom use needs to be separated from contraception. Pregnancy risk factors and HIV/AIDS risk factors are two separate issues, and it appears African American women and men are not making the distinction. This alone may be a major contributor to the escalation of HIV/AIDS among African American women.

African American women cannot afford to be ignorant about the high rate of African American men's HIV infection and risk behaviors. For African American women, the primary way of transmission of the virus is through heterosexual contact. Assumptions and presumptions that your partner is faithful to you or ignorance about past sexual encounters leave women at risk for the virus.

Multiple Partners

There needs to be a deconstruction of two prevailing myths in the African American community: the sex as "taboo" myth and the African American male as "stud" myth. The sex as taboo myth keeps youths and so-called respectable women in denial about their sexual behavior. Youths in a focus group admitted that they did not have multiple partners because that would be a taboo. Their monogamy meant that they were faithful to their partner at the time of the relationship, even if that relationship only lasted 3 weeks (Peeler, 2002). This meant that within a year they could be in four or more monogamous relationships, yet did not see this behavior as multiple partners and risky. African American women tend to think in this vein also. They do not see their behavior as at risk as long as they are only involved with one man at a time. But if these relationships are short-lived and frequent, then this behavior is risky.

The African American male as "stud" myth continues to equate masculine pride and virility with multiple partners. This myth, coupled with refusal to use condoms, exposes not only the African American male but also African American females. African American women are often silent even when they suspect their partner is not faithful because of the shortage of African American men and the old adage that "A piece of man is better than nothing at all." Sharing a man is often seen as the price you pay for being in the African American community. Overby and Kegeles (1994) identified African American adolescent women's lack of recognition of the cumulative importance of both their own and their sexual partners' past sexual relationships as a significant risk factor. Menopausal women are also at risk because they tend to be widowed, divorced, and separated which puts them back in the dating game not really knowing the rules about potential sexual partner's history and the risk factors of HIV/AIDS (HIV/AIDS, 2004).

Research has underscored that not only the issue of multiple partners adds to risk factors for HIV but also the age of the partner, his history, and his age of first engagement in sexual activity. Duberstein et al. (1997) found that older male partners present a greater HIV transmission risk than adolescent males because they are more likely to have had multiple sex partners, to have had varied sexual and drug use experiences, and to be infected with HIV. Duberstein et al. (1997) and Miller et al. (1997) assert that older men engaging in sexual relations with younger women is widespread, but there is a disproportionately high percentage of adult men with minor partners in the African American and Latino communities.

Early sexual engagement is a risk factor in the African American community. Virginity is seen as negative and abstinence as abnormal, and innocence is lost at earlier and earlier ages. Kann et al. (1997) found that among high school students, 11 percent of African American females reported having sexual intercourse by age 13, compared to 3 percent of white females. Over 65 percent of African American female high school students reported having sexual intercourse. These statistics not only add to the high rate of teenage pregnancy and single parenthood in our community, but also promote the escalation of the transmission of HIV in African American females ages 16–34.

Substance abuse (alcohol and other drugs), especially intravenous drug use (IDU) has always been a significant risk factor for transmission of HIV/AIDS in the African American community, but the focus was on the person sharing a needle, not on sexual behavior (multiple partners, lack of condom use, lack of discretion in choosing sexual partners). The Centers for Disease Control (1997) found that nearly 50 percent of all women infected with HIV who contracted it through unprotected sex with an injection drug user and/or a bisexual male are African American. This issue is also directly related to sexual behavior and sexual history. Not only persons who have been intravenous drug users but also other types of chemical abusers engage in irresponsible and high-risk behaviors while under the influence of these substances. Even if the person is in recovery, that history puts them at risk.

Sex and sexuality need to be put in context for the African American community, especially since the media (television, movie, and music industries) continue to bombard our youths and adults with messages of the joys of "promiscuity." Communication about sexual behavior and sexual history is essential, as it relates to high rates of men's HIV infection and risk behaviors. African American women tend to be timid about communication with male partners about their sexual behavior and history. We must get past the "What's your sign?" dialogue of the 1970s and get serious about our health in the twenty-first century. What is needed is open and frank dialogue between African American males and females to address this issue.

Bisexuality among African American Men

Initially, the primary way for the transmission of HIV for African American women was injection drug use. Wingood and DiClemente (1998) reported that 41 percent of the documented AIDS cases for African American women were attributed to injection drug use, but the AIDS cases linked to heterosexual transmission were increasing faster than any other category. The Centers for Disease Control (2003, 2004) have consistently reported that African American women today are primarily infected through sex with men. This means that infection through heterosexual contact has exceeded infection through injection drug use. The implication is that not only a certain class of women are at risk, but all African American women are at high risk.

Many believe that the escalation of HIV transmission to African American women by male-female contact has much to do with African American men being bisexual. There has been a recent focus on African American men who are bisexual, using the slang term men, "on the down-low (DL)." African American gay men, according to Richards (2001) face the double "isms" of racism and sexism, including homophobia, so they negotiate their needs by being on the DL. These men, with a secret sexual lifestyle, fail to disclose their preference for both sexes, and keep their sexual behavior under wraps. The danger is not just the fact that these men are bisexual in their behavior, but according to Richards, the "down-low culture" involves men who call themselves straight but have sexual intercourse with men. Their bisexual behavior is a secret, and African American women are becoming the victims of the coverup.

The unfortunate result is that their clandestine behavior, lack of condom use, and the ignorance of minority heterosexual women about the prevalence of their partners' bisexual behavior has escalated the spread of the disease, especially in the African American community. Brown (2004) calls it dishonesty regarding sexual behavior, which can lead not only to emotional distress but a deadly disease.

Prior to the recent publicizing of the reality of men on the down-low in the Black community, the average woman was clearly uninformed about the probability of her partner engaging in alternative, risky sexual behavior. African American women believed that men who have sex with men are gay. They did not believe that these men might be bisexual. In addition, it is common knowledge in the African American community that men in prison often engage in sex with other men. Before the open discussion of the down-low culture over the past three years, HIV/AIDS services and research had a category called "MSM's— men who have sex with men." This was a distinction between men who were gay and men who may engage in sex with men as the dominant partner, but still had sex with women.

J. L. King has been heralded by the Center for Disease Control on his outspokenness about the down-low culture in the African American community (Christian, 2004). He adamantly distinguishes a man who lives on the down-low from bisexual and homosexual men. He believes that men who are on the DL prefer women, but also enjoy sex with men. He asserts that "D.L. men will never give up the pursuit of having a relationship with a woman because they prefer women over men" (Brown, 2004, p. 86). Unfortunately, King's position appears to support the concept that women should understand and be open to the men who are on the DL, yet should be aware and protect themselves.

Despite King's liberal attitude toward bisexual men, unfortunately, open, intelligent, and loving African American women are being infected, including women who are on all other accounts at low risk for the contraction of the virus. These women do not engage in traditional high-risk behaviors: multiple sex partners, IDU, sex trade, and so on, but they still contract the disease because they are ignorant of the sexual behaviors of their partner and consequently do not see the need to practice safe sex.

Health Literacy

Health and psychological literature concur that African Americans suffer from preventable diseases and premature deaths at a level disproportionately higher than the general population (Thompson & Chambers, 2000). This has been documented especially for hypertension, diabetes, and related kidney failure. It has been suggested that it is true about these diseases because many African Americans are not aware of the link between high blood pressure, diabetes, and kidney disease until they are at the point of dialysis. I believe this lack of awareness and low health literacy is also true for African American women and HIV/AIDS.

The Center for Health Care Strategies (CHCS) asserts that nonwhites and those with low incomes are among the primary populations who are more likely to have trouble reading and understanding health-related information. In addition, CHCS asserts that persons with poor health literacy are more likely to have chronic disease and less likely to receive or seek adequate health care. Unfortunately, health literacy is usually defined as a single factor—trouble reading and understanding health related information. I believe health literacy is a more complex term for African Americans.

During the nineteenth century and first half of the twentieth, the segregated health care system and separate education of health care professionals reflected the attitudes, beliefs, and laws of the majority in a segregated society. For African Americans, mistrust of the American health care system is due to their experience in bondage, folklore, and substantial evidence of exploitation of these individuals during the Tuskegee Syphilis study. In contemporary America, a number of comprehensive studies provide substantial evidence of disparities in health care which may be related to racism and/or bias throughout the spectrum of health care delivery (Watts, 2003).

It is our assumption that in the African American community, health literacy is a more complex issue and that health disparities are maintained in the African American community because of the multiple factors that comprise and influence low health literacy. As it relates to HIV/AIDS and health literacy, there are still many African Americans who believe that the escalation of the disease in the Black community is a conspiracy and fail to take the risk factors seriously. Low health literacy rates combined with cultural mistrust of the health care institutions again put us at risk.

SUMMARY AND CONCLUSION

Health Consciousness and Health Promotion

If safe sexual behavior is the primary way to reduce the incidence of HIV contraction, then this is a worthy goal, but we must reach for it with the awareness that behavioral change can only occur when there is a change in consciousness. I believe that health consciousness and health-promoting behaviors are a new dimension for African Americans in general and especially African American women, who have a history of taking care of everyone and everything else but not themselves.

The disparity between the health status of African Americans and whites has been well documented in medical and social science literature. At all stages of life, men, women, and children of African descent experience more health problems and have more negative outcomes than other cultural groups. It appears that existing health promotion programs have not been successful in reducing the rate of disease and illness among African Americans, overall. In addition, very few of these programs address the psychosocial and sociocultural issues that may contribute to this health disparity.

Thompson and Chambers (2000) discuss the literature regarding health outcomes and African Americans. Their review asserts that researchers have used comparative strategies that contrast African Americans with European Americans on various health-related outcomes. Unfortunately, this strategy has resulted in emphasizing the weaknesses of African Americans rather than strengths. It has also ignored within-group differences. These research approaches, which are widespread not only in health related areas, but generally in social science research, continue to describe African Americans as homogeneous and minimizes the diversity within the group. Because of this monolithic view, African Americans' health status and health behaviors are seen in a limited fashion and health promotion programs implemented by agencies and individuals minimize psychological and sociological structures of the community.

This definitely has been the case with the approach to HIV/AIDS intervention and prevention activities in the African American community. Complex cultural themes prevail and influence, on a group and individual level, how a person will change their behavior as it relates to their health. Thompson and Chambers (2000) propose a relationship between cultural consciousness, health consciousness, and health promoting behaviors for African Americans. Cultural consciousness is the awareness a person has of their cultural identity. Azibo (1996) asserts that psychologists have found that cultural or racial identity is one of the most significant mediators of the African American psychological experience. I believe that this cultural or racial identity for African American women includes the cultural, religious, and gender issues that influence their choices in terms of condom usage and safe sex.

Health consciousness is the degree to which individuals focus on their health through states of attention to self-relevant cues that are reflected in both cognition and affect (Gould, 1990). Gould predicted that health consciousness would relate positively to healthy behaviors and negatively to nonhealthy behaviors. Health-promoting behavior is the extent that a person takes preventive and proactive measures with their health and is attuned to health. This includes eating habits, rest, exercise, protective and prevention activities, and others things that are necessary to preserve a state of optimal physical functioning (Thompson & Chambers, 2000). The formula—cultural consciousness plus health consciousness equals health-promoting behaviors—needs to be applied to intervention and prevention activities.

Prescription for Change

Last, but certainly not the least, involves defining the prescription for change to help arrest the spread of this disease to African American women. The current and most prevalent approach to the problem is behavioral change. First, how do we encourage African American women to, first, become aware that they are at risk, and often at high risk, for HIV/AIDS. Second, once they are aware of this social and physiological phenomenon, how do we move from risky behaviors to safe sex behavior? I believe behavorial change is still the answer, but we must not limit our strategies to only one model of behavior change. We must become broader in our approach and find interventions that fit the complexity of the problem. I believe that once we address these underlying issues, we must not limit our strategies to only one model of behavior change. We must become eclectic in our approach and find interventions that fit the complexity of the problem at hand. DiClemente and Wingood (1995) assert that current models of behavior change have provided useful guidance for understanding HIV risk-reduction practices, but these models have failed to consider a host of contextual social factors that shape the reality of risk and potential risk reduction for African American women.

We must stop minimizing the sociocultural factors (socioeconomic, socio-cultural, psychosocial, sociopolitical, moral, and spiritual) and assess the "real" factors that lead to the escalating levels of infection in the African American community and especially with women. The plain truth is that most of the interventions to arrest the disease in African American communities that are accessible to African Americans tend to mirror strategies that were used for predominantly white and gay communities. The prevailing HIV/AIDS outreach activities that still utilize strategies developed for white gay males, do not, and have not, impacted the HIV/AIDS epidemic in the African American commu-nity. In addition, interventions that focus just on African American women are very few in number. Evidently, interventions that are not founded on quality research and insight into the true nature of the target population, and only replicate interventions for Euro-Americans, will not help us to retard the spread of the disease.

One issue that stands out for me in terms of developing a prescriptive focus for this population is the fact that safe sex does not appear to be a high priority for African American women. The use of condoms today is no longer aimed at contraception. It is primarily promoted as a way to protect your health and your life. It appears that African American women, for a variety of reasons have not made this transition in consciousness and behavior about the different use of the condom.

If the focus of behavorial change and prevention for HIV/AIDS is focused on condom use only, and African American women are not utilizing this strategy, we must find out why. What are the blockages in consciousness that keeps us from embracing this strategy and utilizing health-promoting behaviors? I believe we need to consider the formula, cultural consciousness plus health conscious-ness equals health promoting behaviors, and apply it to intervention and pre-vention activities for African American women. The cultural consciousness aspect for African American women includes not only the racial issues but the gender issues. I also believe health promotion for African American women must include the psychological aspect that includes a look at Maslow's hierarchy

(Maslow, 1943). Apparently, African American women continue in risky behavior or denial about their at-risk status because they assert their social needs above their survival and safety needs. Health consciousness is safety and survival. Health-promoting behaviors for African American women, as they relate to HIV/AIDS, must address these social issues and analyze how we think and what we believe, if we are going to address this epidemic in our community and save lives.

Final Thoughts

I began this chapter with some descriptive words: epidemic, pandemic, endemic, disproportionate, escalation, and epicenter. These words are ominous as it relates to African American women but the greater issue is how and what do we do to arrest and be proactive in reducing the incidence and prevalence of the disease in our community and among African American women. I believe that more psychosocial research needs to done to develop prevention and intervention activities that address the specific needs of African American women. This research needs to factor in the cultural and gender issues, as well as, how African American women can help themselves and their other African sisters in the diaspora who are also being victimized by HIV/AIDS. Plain talk will get us moving, and the plain truth will save us.

REFERENCES

Azibo, D. A. 1996. "Personality, Clinical, and Social Psychological Research on 'Blacks': Appropriate and Inappropriate Research Frameworks." In D. A. Azibo (Ed.), *African Psychology in Historial Perspective and Related Commentary*, pp. 203–234. Trenton, NJ: Africa World Press.

Brown, J. F. October 2004. "J. L. King's Graphic Story of Life as a Man on the Down Low." *Sistah 2 Sistah*.

Centers for Disease Control and Prevention. 1997. *HIV/AIDS Surveillance Report* 9(1): 1–39.

———. Division of HIV/AIDS Prevention. 2002. *HIV/AIDS Surveillance Report: Midyear Edition, U.S. HIV and AIDS Cases Reported through June 2002*.

———. Division of HIV/AIDS Prevention. 2003. *HIV/AIDS among African Americans— Fact Sheet*. Available online at http://www.cdc.gov/hiv/pubs/facts/afam.htm.

Christian, M. A. 2004. "Men on the Down Low: Author J. L. King Exposes the Sex Secret That Is Devastating Black Women." *Jet* 105(18):32–37.

DiClemente, R. J. 1992. "African Americans and AIDS: Confronting the Challenge of AIDS in the African-American Community." *Ethnicity & Disease* 2, 358–60.

DiClemente, R. J., and G. M. Wingwood. 1995. "A Randomized Controlled Trial of an HIV Sexual Risk-reduction Intervention for Young African-American Women." *Journal of American Medical Association* 274, no. 16.

Duberstein, L. L., F. L. Sonenstein, L. Ku, et al. 1997. "Age Differences between Minors Who Give Birth and Their Adult Partners." *Family Planning Perspectives* 2, 61–66.

Gould, S. J. 1990. Health Consciousness and Health Behaviors: The Application of a New Health Consciousness Scale. *American Journal of Preventive Medicine* 6(4):228–37.

Guttentag, M., and P. F. Secord. 1983. *Too Many Women? The Sex Ratio Question.* Beverly Hills, CA: Sage Publishers.

Haverkos, H. W., F. Turner, Jr., E. T. Moolchan, and J. L. Cadet. 1999. "Relative Rates of AIDS among Racial/Ethnic Groups by Exposure Categories." *Journal of National Medicine Association* 91(1):17–24.

Hearn, K. D., and L. R. Jackson. 2002. "African American Women and HIV Risk: Exploring the Effects of Gender and Social Dynamics on Behavior." *African American Research Perspectives* 8(1), 163–173.

HIV/AIDS: People of Color and Women. 2004. *Senior Health Newsletter.* Available online at http://Seniorhealthabout.com/library/sex/blaids4.htm.

Jones, C., and K. Shorter-Gooden. 2003. *Shifting: The Double Lives of Black Women in America.* New York: HarperCollins Publishers.

Kann, L., S. A. Kinchen, B. I. Williams, J. G. Ross, J. A. Grunbaum, and L. J. Kolbe, 1997. "Youth Risk Behavior Surveillance." *Journal of School Health* 70(7): 271–285.

Kimberly, J. A., and J. M. Serovich. 1999. *The Role of Family and Friend Social Support in Reducing Risk Behaviors among HIV Positive Gay Men.* New York: Guilford Publishing.

King, J. L. 2004. *On the Down Low: A Journey into the Lives of "Straight" Black Men Who Sleep with Men.* New York: Broadway Books.

Maslow, A. H. 1943. "A Theory of Human Motivation." *Psychological Review* 50, 370–396.

McNair, L. D., and C. M. Prather. 2004. "African American Women and AIDS: Factors Influencing Risk and Reaction to HIV Disease." *Journal of Black Psychology* 30(1):106–23.

Miller, K. S., et al. 1997. "Sexual Initiation with Older Male Partners and Subsequent Behavior among Female Adolescents." *Family Planning Perspectives* 29, 21.

National Institute of Health. 2003. Addressing Health Disparities. The NIH Program of Action. Available online at http://healthdisparities.nih.gov/faqs.html.

New York State AIDS Advisory Council. Winter 2000/2001. *Communities at Risk: HIV/AIDS in Communities of Color.*

Overby, K. J., and S. M. Kegeles. 1994. "The Impact of AIDS On an Urban Population of High-risk Female Minority Adolescents: Implications For Intervention." *Journal of Adolescent Health* 15, 216–27.

Peeler, L. E. 2002. *Sex, Lies and Social Constructions: HIV-Related Knowledge, Attitudes and Behaviors of African-Americans in Buffalo, New York—2000 Sample.* Buffalo, NY: Prominent Life Resources.

Pittman, K. J., P. M. Wilson, S. Adams-Taylor, et al. 1992. "Making Sexuality Education and Prevention Programs Relevant for African American Youth." *Journal of School Health* 62, 339–44.

Richards, Diane. 2001. "AIDS Campaign Focuses on the 'Down Low.'" *Contemporary Sexuality* 35, 6.

Roberson, N. L. 1996. "Exploring Health Issues and Health Status of African American Women with Emphasis on Cancer." In C. F. Collins (Ed.), *African American Women's Health and Social Issues.* Westport, CT: Praeger.

Thompson, S. N., and J. W. Chambers, Jr. 2000. "African Self-Consciousness and Health Promoting Behaviors among African American College Students." *Journal of Black Psychology* 26(3):300–345.

U.S. Census Bureau. March 1999. *The Black Population in the United States*. Current Population Survey.

Washington, E. D., Jr. 2000. "Knowing, Believing, and Understanding: The Social Construction of Knowledge in the O.J. Simpson Criminal Trial." *Journal of Black Psychology* 26(3):302–16.

Watts, Rosalyn J. 2003. "Race Consciousness and the Health of African Americans." *Journal of Issues in Nursing*. Available online at http://www.nursing.upenn.

Williams, P. B., O. Keundayo, and I. Udezulu. 2003. "An Ethnically Sensitive and Gender-Specific HIV/AIDS Assessment of African American Women: A Comparative Study of Urban and Rural American Communities." *Family Community Health* 26(2):108–24.

Wingood, G. M., and R. J. DiClemente. 1997. "Consequences of Having a Physically Abusive Partner on the Condom Use and Sexual Negotiation Practices of Young Adult African-American Women." *American Journal of Public Health* 87, 1016–18.

———. 1998. "Pattern Influences and Gender Related Factors Associated with Noncondom Use among Young Adult African American Women." *American Journal of Community Psychology* 26, 29–49.

Wingood, G. M., R. J. DiClemente, D. H. McCree, K. Harrington, and S. L. Davies. 2001. "Dating Violence and the Sexual Health of Black Adolescent Females." *Pediatrics* 5(107):72. Available online at http://pediatrics.aappublications.org/cgi/content/full/107/5/e72.

Wyatt, G. E., N. G. Forge, and D. Guthrie. 1998. "Family Constellation and Ethnicity: Current and Lifetime HIV-Related Risk Taking." *Journal of Family Psychology* 1(12):93–101.

7

Social Construction
and Social Transmission
of HIV/AIDS

LORRAINE E. PEELER

Statistics about human immunodeficiency virus/acquired immunodeficiency syndrome (HIV/AIDS) indicate that African American men and women are ten times more likely to acquire AIDS from a heterosexual relationship than a same sex relationship. In addition, African American women are at 10 to 15 times greater risk of HIV infections than Euro-American women. Unfortunately, the average African American woman is not aware of these statistical facts. In addition, the majority of the research literature on African American women and HIV/AIDS focuses on persons who are economically disadvantaged and ages 18–44 years old. It does not address the full range of African American women, regardless of social class, age, and education. I believe there is a gap in research, and consequently, culturally sensitive interventions, because there is a lack of understanding about African American culture. This puts the whole spectrum of African American women at risk of the virus.

Please note that there is a difference between high risk and at risk. A high-risk person is a person who is directly exposed to the virus due to documented lifestyle. For example, if you or your significant other are intravenous drug users or share needles, if you have sex without the use of condoms and with multiple partners, or if you are a sex trade worker, you are in the high-risk category. The at-risk person is the person who is indirectly exposed. You could be engaging in an assumed monogamous relationship, not using condoms, not aware of the chemical dependence pattern, bisexual lifestyle, or multiple partners of your partner, or you may just be ignorant to the reality of HIV/AIDS in your community.

The discussion of HIV/AIDS in the African American community leaves the door open for many unanswered questions. Some questions are: Why has HIV/ AIDS become such a threat in the African American community? Why are African American women the fastest growing group that is being infected with the virus? Why are African American women and most of the African American community not aware that this is the case? Why are there not culturally sensitive and culturally competent interventions designed to arrest this disease in our communities? I believe the answers to these questions are revealed in one conceptual answer—HIV/AIDS is not just a sexually transmitted disease but a socially transmitted disease. This conceptualization, of HIV/AIDS as a socially transmitted disease, is what places African American women more at risk, and, in many instances, at high risk, for the virus.

It is necessary to address the impact of HIV/AIDS in the African American population from a social psychological perspective to address the complexity of the disease in our community and go beyond the use of condoms, to deeper aspects that confront, not only our behaviors, but the internal motivators of those behaviors. There is also a definite intersection of different variables that influence African American women and the potential of contracting HIV/AIDS, which is different for African American men and for Euro-American women.

African American women are increasingly at risk because there is not a straight line between our potential exposure to the disease and issues that complicate health-promoting behaviors. Specifically, social structure and societal stereotypes are part of the social construction of HIV/AIDS in the African American community. The complexity of this disease impacts some fundamental issues that go beyond our sexual behavior and delves into the motivators of our behaviors that ignore warning signs and caution lights, as well as clear and present dangers. It deals with our myths, stereotypes, lies, and taboos related to our sexual life, our sexuality, and our social psychological beliefs, as well as gender issues and racial trauma.

Why is our social psychology important? Social psychology is the science that seeks to understand the nature and cause of individual behavior and thought in social situations. This includes attitudes and beliefs and how they motivate behavior. It focuses on the behavior of individuals and seeks to understand the causes of social behavior and thought. Consequently, as we confront the important perspective that HIV/AIDS is not only a sexually transmitted disease, but also a socially transmitted disease, the contraction of the virus has psychological implications. The literature implies that African American women are at high risk of HIV infection due to risk behaviors they may engage in. These risk behaviors are not only sexually motivated but also socially motivated and related to their social psychological perspectives in the society, which includes the influence of culture and racio-ethnic identity.

Social construction is also an important aspect of understanding the relationship between HIV/AIDS and African Americans' risk factors. Social construction is an interdisciplinary concept that draws from numerous sources: sociology, literary study, history, anthropology, women's studies, psychology, communication, cultural studies, and more (Gergen, 2001). Gergen asserts that the critique that social constructionists bring to the academic disciplines appeals to marginalized groups and those who are in pursuit of social equality and justice.

Social construction theory gives a voice to these groups across disciplines. Social construction has a place in psychology and in a further explanation of social psychological impact. Gergen believes there is no antagonism between psychology and social construction. He asserts that psychology adds to the "social reconstitution" of the individual and gives significant attention to "language, dialogue, negotiation, social pragmatics, conversational positioning, ritual, cultural practice and the distribution of power" (Gergen, 2001, p. 37). The relationship between social construction and psychology includes individuals as cultural carriers; individuals are culturally immersed and influenced by their relationships with others.

In addition to race and/or ethnicity as a risk factor, psychological and sociological variables including attitudes, and in particular attitudes toward gay men and lesbians, have contributed to the social construction of HIV/AIDS as a stigmatized disease. In other words, responses to prevention and intervention are further challenged due to an association with groups that are already stigmatized by society.

If this is true, then in order to understand the relationship between African American women and the transmission of HIV/AIDS to this group, we must understand them as cultural carriers who are immersed in their culture and influenced by their relationships, especially with the opposite sex. In addition, this social construction is complicated by the symbolic meaning of HIV/AIDS in the African American culture, which is negative because the initial reports regarding HIV/AIDS, describe and allude to a perception of the disease as impacting persons who are socially deviant and support a certain lifestyle, a group that includes white homosexual and bisexual men (DiClemente, 1992; Kimberly & Serovich, 1999).

It is necessary to understand not just how African Americans socially construct the disease, but also how other groups socially construct African Americans. More often than not, African Americans are socially constructed as pathological, undeserving, unintelligent, and deviant. Not only do social constructions constitute negative images, beliefs, and values about culturally oppressed groups, but, DiClemente (1992) asserts, such constructions have led to the interplay between African Americans and increasing numbers of HIV/AIDS transmissions. He believes a person's behavior (particularly, the lack of appropriate HIV prevention behaviors) propels the epidemic. In other words, HIV/AIDS is considered a sexual (biological) and behavioral (social) problem that identifies a specific race and/or ethnicity (cultural) as one of the major risk factors for contracting the disease (Lester, 1993). Therefore, the perpetuation of fear among African Americans to talk openly and freely about HIV/AIDS hampers interventions as well as prevents others from gaining the information necessary to keep themselves and their community free of this disease.

SOCIAL CONSTRUCTION OF CONDOM USE

Physical factors have been identified that may be responsible for the increase of HIV/AIDS transmission to African American women, which centers on the lack of condom use, but apparently, for various reasons, this intervention has not been effective. Our focus is to look at the psychosocial factors that have impacted the epidemic for women. McNair and Prather (2004) summarize factors that are directly related to HIV risks and African American women on two dimensions: social and contextual. Social factors are variables that impact groups of people similarly but are external to the individuals, like cultural beliefs, values, and practices. Contextual factors are variables that are environmental aspects that influence an individual's perspective and therefore have import only for that person, such as relationship history, victimization experience, and levels of environmental stress.

The literature supports the hypothesis that social factors are predominant variables in why there is such a high rate of contraction of HIV/AIDS among African American women. McNair and Prather (2004) identify four social factors that are unique to the HIV/AIDS epidemic as it relates to African American women. What makes these factors unique is that the exposure for the women is through heterosexual contact. These social factors are: (1) the sex-ratio imbalance, (2) low levels of condom use, (3) high rates of men's HIV infection and risk behaviors, and (4) lack of disclosure regarding bisexuality among African American men. In Chapter 6, I address all of these issues. To address the social transmission focus, I would like to focus on the low levels of condom use, because this intervention is still pushed as the main factor that will reduce the transmission, yet it has not yielded the results in the African American community, and especially for African American women. The sex-ratio imbalance, multiple partners, bisexuality, and other all culminate in non–condom use.

My focus HIV/AIDS as a social disease, will center on the lack of condom use by African American women and the proposed reasons why the "safe sex" message does not cut across the barriers of attitudes and beliefs. Some of the proposed reasons include: personal, relational, and social roles; gender equity, cultural, and religious aspects; denial and social construction of non–condom use.

Low Levels of Condom Use

For African American women, the low levels of condom use are a documented fact and a complex issue. The fact that African American women contract HIV/ AIDS at an alarming rate is evidence that "safe sex" is not a priority. Although safe sex is the buzzword in prevention strategies in the gay community, it is not a priority in the African American community, and there is a need to examine why and what factors are essential to reducing the risk for sexually active African American women. We need to confront and examine factors associated with non–condom use during sexual intercourse in this population, from the psychosocial perspective.

Various studies (DiClemente & Wingood, 1995; McNair & Prather, 2004) report a high rate of non–condom use for African American women for a variety of reasons that include: perceived inconvenience of using condoms, which can block spontaneity; perceived negative impact of using condoms on sexual enjoyment, especially as reported by their male partner; and the belief that using condoms negatively impacts relationship trust. Participants in these studies report that if they ask their partner to use a condom, there is an implication that the partner is engaging in sexual activity with others.

If the rate of contraction of HIV/AIDS is the highest in the country for African American women, then we must make a direct correlation that a significant portion of these women consistently engage in unprotected sex. If they are continuing to engage in unprotected sex based on perceptions and beliefs (social psychology and social construction), then we need to understand and address the power of perceptions and beliefs. Interventions need to be made on that level.

Johnson et al. (1994) suggest that lack of awareness of the causes and routes of transmission of HIV/AIDS is responsible for the alarming increase in the disease among this group. Their research asserted that there were some other potential factors, which included: lack of knowledge and incorrect attitudes about AIDS; emotional reactions toward condom use; distinct attitudes toward the role of condoms in a sexual encounter; risky sexual behaviors (i.e., anal intercourse, sex with multiple partners, sex with prostitutes or persons who sleep with prostitutes, drug use). This research is significant because it outlined some important and often overlooked issues like attitudes.

Johnson et al. (1994) used a sample of 304 African Americans and 104 whites. Some of the findings highlighted unrealistic expectations about relationships and fidelity. Specifically, a significant percentage in both groups felt that a condom was not necessary if you loved your partner. High-risk sexual behaviors were also identified, and a racial difference between the types of risky behaviors was prevalent. More whites than Blacks reported engaging in anal sex and more Blacks than whites reported having sex with prostitutes. Blacks perceived themselves to be at greater risk for contracting HIV than whites, although safe sex behaviors were not greater for that group, despite their perceptions of the risk factors.

Attitudes about the use of condoms did not differ between African Americans and whites, but Johnson et al. (1994) found that African Americans experienced a significantly greater "intense angry" reaction during the negotiation and use of condoms than did the white subjects. The researchers suggest that the intensity of anger surrounding the use of condoms in the African American populations may be interfering with the rational decision to protect oneself from the consequences of risky sex.

Personal, Relational, and Social Roles

I believe the finding of the anger reaction in itself is significant to African American women and HIV/AIDS. The use of condoms today is no longer aimed at contraception. It is primarily promoted as a way to protect your health and your life. The anger identified by African American men appears to be due to three distinct areas: personal, relational, and social roles. The personal aspect has to do with making an assumption about the partner's health status. If a woman asks a man about his HIV or STD status, it is a personal indictment about his health, and health is a personal issue. If you also ask a man to use a condom, it represents assuming that the man is unclean and/or unhealthy.

The relational aspect is based on the insinuation of infidelity in the relationship. If the woman asks a man to use a condom and they are in an assumed monogamous relationship, the use of a condom represents mistrust. The social role aspect is based on the shifting of the balance of power or control in the relationship. It is implied that if the man makes the choice about a condom, it is okay—but if the woman makes the choice or asserts her need for the use of the condom, she is asserting power. Condom use initiated by a woman implies a gender equity position. Johnson et al.'s (1994) research found that even though men engaged in more risky sexual practices, it was the men who were more likely to always use condoms. This suggests that men are making the decisions regarding the use of condoms in the sexual arena, and they believe this is their right and not the right of the woman.

The impact of these beliefs and perceptions for African American women and their relationships with men are life-threatening. A study by Overby and Kegeles (1994) of African American women ages 13 to 19 found that 26 percent felt they had little control over whether a condom is used during intercourse. Moreover, 75 percent agreed that if a male partner knows that the woman is taking oral contraceptives, the male will not want to use a condom. A majority of this sample believed that a male sex partner would be hurt, insulted, angry, or suspicious if questioned about his HIV risk factors. Other studies of African American women found that there is a direct relationship between relationship violence and adverse sexual health behaviors (Wingood & DiClemente, 1997; Wingood et al., 2001). Overall, women usually take responsibility for contraception but often do not insist on using contraception if they fear abuse (Wyatt, 1997). This abuse could be physical or emotional, especially if men display intense anger when asked to use a condom.

The issue is that condom use needs to be separated from contraception. Pregnancy-risk factors and HIV/AIDS risk factors are two separate issues, and it appears African American women and men are not making the distinction. This in itself may be a major contributor to the escalation of HIV/AIDS among African American women. Thus, it is vital to identify the psychosocial, relational, and gender-related factors associated with African American women's non–condom use.

Gender Equity

The three components identified as personal, relational, and social roles are important variables to confront and investigate as they relate to African American women's health and risk of contracting HIV/AIDS. All three directly impact these women's health and how they will respond to interventions and behavioral change. However, two out of the three issues have to do with the gender equity and deserves further discussion. These gender equity issues need to be addressed, especially when the average African American woman, influenced by Judeo-Christian as well as Islamic ethics, still views the man, whether the husband or a significant other, as the "head of the house." This conceptualization of power has left African American women vulnerable.

Gender-related dynamics are powerful and include the man as the head of the household, gender roles and power roles used in intimate relationships, managing interpersonal relationships, and their relationship to risk reduction practices (Bowleg et al., 2000). Bowleg and colleagues believe that gender role orientation for African American women is extremely complex because sexual identity and gender role orientation may operate as independent personality dimensions. Lester (1993) speaks to this complexity and believes that factors that are related to gender are compounded by race, economic circumstances, and powerlessness, which contributes to psychosocial victimization. Some people have termed the plight of African American women as "multiple jeopardy," referring to the interaction of class, race, and gender.

Hearn and Jackson (2002) believe that socialization and concepts of femininity and masculinity are a part of these general related dynamics, which influence the sexual health of African American women and underscore the male-dominant and female-subordinate gender roles in the African American community. This is often played out to mean that women are expected to be sexually naive and men sexually astute. Johnson et al. (1994) assert that the women in their sample had more knowledge about AIDS than men but still continued to participate in potentially risky practices and relinquished the responsibility of their own health to the male.

Jones and Shorter-Goodman (2003) believe African American women shift to the point that they cushion their men and endanger their own health. They call them "Sisterellas," which is defined as depressed Black women who silence themselves and shift into hyper-performance, largely to protect and support their men. I believe that these women endanger their own health, not only emotionally but also physically, just in the name of maintaining the relationship and not upsetting the balance of power in the relationship; in short, they give their power away. In contrast, Hearn and Jackson (2002) assert that historically the relationship between African American men and women has been more balanced due to societal barriers against Black men. They believe that because African American women contribute to the household, they have some degree of influence in the household. This may be true about household matters, but it has not played out in the areas of sexuality.

For African American women the gender-related factors are confounded by cultural factors, and both are interlaced with religious values and morality issues. The myth of the "strong Black woman" or the "Black Matriarch" has given African American women a false sense of their coping abilities. Jones and Shorter-Goodman (2003) state that it is a supreme irony that Black women, who are mythologized and relied on for their strength, so often have to submerge their savvy and fortitude to make their partners feel at ease (p. 208). The "strong Black women" syndrome is more of a position of compromise in the face of multiple jeopardy involving the pressures of race, class, and gender.

African American women are socialized to make their partners feel "like a man," while they suppress their own knowledge, wisdom, and expertise. The stereotypical African American woman portrayed in media is a feisty, loud-talking, no-nonsense person. Many Black women are this way on the outside, but on the inside they have more than their share of insecurities, fears, and demons. They might even remain true to the stereotype to their outside friends and families, but when they are with their man, they want to be the feminine, soft person that they are, and this is the part of them that is vulnerable in their intimate relationships. Jones and Shorter-Goodman assert from their research that African American women are often forced to shift in intimate relationships with Black men, sublimating their own needs, strengths, and desires. They found that many Black women feel pressured to reduce their directness and assertiveness and minimize their accomplishments and success to make the men in their lives comfortable with them and confident in their own manhood.

Gender issues have to do with issues of power and control. When you relinquish your power to another person, you are saying that, in the name of love, companionship, or a sexual relationship, someone else knows what is best for you. These power differential issues influence women's ability to make informed decisions. It is demonstrated in their failure to communicate their needs on many levels, especially as they relate to their health. Issues related to gender and power differences lend strong support for the needs for HIV/AIDS interventions that empower African American women to take a greater responsibility for minimizing risky sexual behavioral practices.

Race, Culture, and Religion

The research is consistent that non–condom use and other gender-related issues, especially power differentials and relationship/communication variables, affect the mind-set that is necessary to move African American women toward behavioral change. For African American women these variables are compounded by imbedded cultural and religious issues. Intervention and prevention activities must be developed and implemented to address these insidious and subtle elements that influence African American women's choices.

Unfortunately, the Centers for Disease Control do see race and/or ethnicity as a risk factor, and African Americans, especially women, are disproportionately infected by the disease. Hearn and Jackson (2002) believe that for African American women there is an interplay of race, gender, age, and class that makes them particularly at risk. Since the early 1990s, DiClemente et al. (1992, 1993, 1995) have highlighted the need for culturally competent, socially contextual, and gender-based interventions.

In this context I combine culture with the religious aspect, because it is in this interplay between religion and culture that gender beliefs and issues are cultivated and reinforced. There is a strong relationship between cultural beliefs and the "Black Church," which has had a long-term influence on sociocultural belief systems. Betsch Cole and Guy-Sheftall (2003), in their ground-breaking book entitled *Gender Talk: The Struggle for Women's Equality in African American Communities*, address this relationship and its impact in the lives of African American men and women. They state:

We were struck by the fact that every woman and man who participated in the multilogue at the Ford Foundation continued to reference the Black church even if they were no longer members of a particular congregation. This widespread association of Black folks with "the Church" means that centuries-old patterns of patriarchal attitudes and behavior could continue. Or, ideally, these institutions to which millions of Black people are attached in varying degrees could become sites for the transformation of fundamental ideas and values about gender. (p. 127)

I am a product of the cultural/religious tradition of the African American community, and know too well the rhetoric of "the man is the head of the household," regardless of his inability to lead, protect and/or be faithful. In this tradition, the woman who is assertive, who has had to raise her family alone, or who is single is not supported or encouraged. The encouragement is to get or find a man, and that will validate you. Women in the Black Church are encouraged to submit to their husbands. Submission is a popular word in the Black Church and is often defined as the woman obeying her husband without question. Jones and Shorter-Goodman (2003) call it "dangerous submission" that African American women do in their romantic relationships, term it an open door for violence and abuse on multiple levels. It is interesting that an institution like the Black Church, that has been heralded for its activism in terms of racial equality and liberation, keeps its head in the sand on issues of sexism, equality, and liberation for women.

Betsch Cole and Guy-Sheftall (2003) believe that communication, or what they call "gender talk" is an essential component of any intervention and must include spiritual and religious leaders. I believe it must also include interventions that address the spiritual and religious beliefs that have been enmeshed with our cultural norms. This communication must be presented in a way that it does not destroy faith, but rather clarifies the truth that will set women free to protect themselves and their futures. Betsch Cole and Guy-Sheftall assert that this gender talk, or plain talk as I like to call it, is a prerequisite to a consciousness that will lead to behavioral change and impact the lives of women physically, spiritually, and sexually.

Consequently, gender roles and norms in the African American community cannot be separated from the cultural/religious context. There is a definite enmeshment between the three—culture, religion, and gender roles. Any intervention that keeps them separate and distinct does not impact the complexities of the African American woman's attitudes and beliefs.

Jones and Shorter-Goodman (2003), in their book entitled *Shifting: The Double Lives of Black Women in America*, do an excellent job of presenting the complexities of being African American and a woman in America. Gender theory rarely incorporates the interactive effects of race, ethnicity, and culture. Although important, it is based on the experiences of Euro-American women in this society and therefore leaves out key elements in the experience of African American women. African American women have the issues of beauty, which includes the predominant image of beauty in the media as a Euro-American woman, as well as within-group issues of beauty that have to do with skin color and length and type of hair. There are also expectations of size and shape as compared to Euro-American women.

Jones and Shorter-Goodman (2003) devote a chapter to the issues of Black women and beauty and Black women and men. They believe that the core issue in the relationship between African American women and men is the women's attempt to forge a delicate balance in the face of a racist and unfriendly society. The difficulty of relationships for African American couples include: dealing with the impact of racism; gauging how much liberation is okay for a woman; managing competition in the relationship; beauty and image; submission that can lead to violence and abuse; and managing their sexuality in the face of the HIV epidemic (Jones & Shorter-Gooden, 2003).

Denial

On some level, African American women must be in denial about their vulnerability to the disease, despite their knowledge of it. Denial is defined, from a psychological perspective, as an unconscious defense mechanism characterized by refusal to acknowledge the painful realities of a situation. Part of the denial could have to do with the sex-ratio imbalance. The fact is that most African American women believe the availability of men is limited, so when they are engaged in a relationship, they are more compliant and less demanding because of the shortage.

On the other hand, many economically disadvantaged African Americans believe that they have a limited range of pleasures due to their socioeconomic status. Sexual activity remains as one of the few pleasures they have control over. To introduce the boundaries imposed by the fear of contracting HIV/AIDS robs this pleasure of its spontaneity and transforms it into a cognitive activity that takes forethought and is to be entered into with much trepidation.

This denial aspect also relates to the research on lack of condom use by African Americans. Johnson et al. (1994) discusses the anger displayed by African American men during the negotiation and use of condoms in the sexual relationship. I believe this angry reaction is more frustration than anger. The frustration is in response to the new boundaries and cognitions that have now been introduced into what used to be an activity that was spontaneous and designed for pleasure, not deep thought and negotiation. The women concede to non–condom use because they want the man to stay or return. The denial of the realities of the probability that they could be infected and the complexity of engaging in sexual activities (lack of spontaneity), could serve as a block to any knowledge acquired that could lead to behavior change.

Denial is an attitude of feigned ignorance. Attitudes are beliefs and feelings that can influence our reactions and behaviors. The pretense of ignorance, negative feelings about HIV/AIDS, and boundaries imposed by prevention activities apparently influences the lack of preventive behavior for African American women. In addition, this pretense of ignorance is coupled with surprise that the disease is an epidemic in their community and that the probability that they would encounter someone that is infected is high.

Social Construction of Non–Condom Use

Wingood and DiClemente (1998) explored the partner influences and gender-related relationship of non–condom use among low-income and middle-income young adult African American women. This research was grounded in the theory of gender and power, which includes the sexual division of labor, power, and how African American women invest meaning into these areas. They also examined how they socially construct the meaning of their relationship with men.

They purport that condom use is socially constructed and the use of the condom has deeper meanings than "safe sex." The significance implied by the use of a condom is based on the specific woman, but for African American women, they assert the meanings include:

* sexually availability
* compromising traditional religious values
* blocking conception, if interested in having children (the woman or her partner)
* undermining the trust in the relationship
* blocking enjoyment in sex from the male and/or female perspective
* blocking the ability to land a man especially when the pool of eligible men is limited

Consequently, the use of the condom means more than simply safe sex and/or protection from HIV. For example, the social construction of carrying a condom, insisting that your partner use a condom, and consistently using a condom has a multiple impact. For a woman to carry condoms in her purse could suggest that she is available for sex, free with her body, and/or ready for action with whoever asks. A woman who insists that her partner use a condom, especially if they are in a committed relationship, is making a statement about the commitment of her partner or his health status. A woman who only has sex with men who wear condoms may believe that she limits her chances of having children. If that is important to her or her partner, she may not insist that he do so. Last, if a woman believes the pool of eligible men is limited and she also believes that she has to compete with other women, she may also believe that if she insists on the use of a condom and he does not want to use one, he may move on to other women who will not insist.

The literature indicates that social constructions shape beliefs and attitudes and manifest itself in behavior that is either positive (preventive measures) or negative (risky) (DiClemente, 1992; Bradford & Kennamer, 1995). Identifying community morals, values, and beliefs may contribute toward understanding African American women's processing of knowledge and implementation of behaviors within a social context. According to DiClemente (1992) and DiClemente and Wingood (1998), although the knowledge base about HIV/AIDS has expanded for African American women, some social constructions continue to shape their views inaccurately about this disease. These social constructions are influenced by gender roles, issues, the lack of available African American men, and the risky behaviors of the men they open themselves to. To this end, HIV/AIDS is as much a sociocultural phenomenon as it is a biological phenomenon.

This social construction also impacts social/moral issues and women's ability to communicate their health promotion needs. For example, I assisted in conducting a focus group with ten women who had been diagnosed with HIV or had been exposed to the virus. Specific questions were asked and dialogue ensued. One issue that came up in the focus group was the practice of safe sex and the need to be balanced and honest in their approach to it. Many of the women talked about celibacy as a way to practice safe sex and said abstinence was in line with their religious beliefs. They disclosed that maintaining celibacy was a challenge and in the times when they were not celibate, they divulged, they did not practice safe sex for various reasons: spontaneous sexual encounter or admission of guilt based on religious or moral convictions. Abstinence sounded good in theory but did not necessarily play out in practice or encourage wise choices in terms of safe sex.

I believe this social construction is extremely important to identifying some of the underlying variables that keep African American women from making healthy choices. How African American women socially construct their relationship to the men in their lives includes the norms and social rules about sexual behavior, as well as the lack of self-esteem that comes from their racial and cultural identity and their gender identity in this country.

Williams et al. (2003) conducted a comparative study of urban and rural African American women with a focus on ethnically sensitive and gender-specific issues. They utilized the social cognitive theory, health belief model, and the transtheoretical model of behavior change to design an approach and attempt to explain behaviors. They believe that the epidemic nature of the HIV infection among African American women underscores the females' physical, emotional, and sociocultural vulnerability to HIV/AIDS. The surprising findings from this research was the high level of negative attitudes, feelings, mistrusts, and misconceptions of the subjects (81.6 percent of the rural homes), who generally believed that HIV/AIDS among African Americans was part of a "governmental genocidal plot" against the Black race. They associated it with historically documented incidents like the Tuskegee experiment and the sterilization of many African American women without their knowledge.

Thus, among some African Americans, persistent inequality, despair, and painful memories of medical abuses and the consequent anger and mistrust of the U.S. government have contributed to conspiracy theories that hamper HIV education. Mistrust of the government and the health care and social services systems is part of imbedded cultural beliefs and can block prevention and training efforts.

Hearn and Jackson (2002) believe that only by overcoming the multiple barriers that hamper the ability of African American women to make healthy decision about their lives will the spread of HIV decline and the effects of the epidemic be reduced among this population. If the risk factors for African American women are compounded by additional variables, we need to explore the complexity of the issues. What are some potential issues that need to be addressed to help move us toward the necessary behavioral changes that will save the lives of African American women? Let us address some of the issues that must become a part of the intervention strategies to address the epidemic.

PREVENTION AND INTERVENTION STRATEGIES

Plain Talk—Plain Truth

A plain talk means we need to address the plain truth. The plain truth is that African American women across age, education, and socioeconomic levels are at risk and high risk for infection of HIV/AIDS. The plain truth is that despite traditional prevention and intervention methods, the rate for infection for African American women has continued to escalate. The plain truth is that African American women are at risk by way of heterosexual relationships more than through injection drug use. The plain truth is that the rates are only going to decrease once African American women confront and get honest about the mind-sets and behaviors that leave them at risk for this deadly disease.

The apparent truth is that a multitude of prevention and interventions have been employed in our communities and yet the epidemic disproportionately impacts African American women. Obviously, despite the success of these interventions in other communities, they are not effective in our community. The question is why? Why is the message not getting through to African American women to a degree that we see behavioral change and the reduction of the transmission?

The obvious issue is condom use and the practice of safe sex. The facts are in that consistent condom use is the most effective prevention for the transmission of HIV. The statistics underscore the alarming fact that significant and disproportionate numbers of African American women do not actively practice safe sex. But condom use and the practice of safe sex are behavioral issues. This presupposes that there must be confounding social psychological variables that are not being addressed in current prevention and intervention methodologies that block behavioral change for African American men and women. Evidently, these attitudes and beliefs are so strong and imbedded that African American women risk their lives for them. Consequently, there is a desperate need to identify them and develop appropriate interventions to help the women overcome them.

Let us revisit the need to address the social psychology of African American women. The prevention and intervention literature and activities focus on knowledge, attitudes, beliefs and behaviors (KABB), but the message is still predominantly condom use. We need to have interventions that not only address our behaviors but our thoughts that lead us to these behaviors. What are the behaviors and thoughts on a social and individual level that lead us to risky behavior and loss of health? This focus must be emphasized because HIV/AIDS is not only a sexually transmitted disease, it is also a socially transmitted disease and contraction has psychological implications. If the disease is socially transmitted through our sexual behaviors, if the social interaction that has us at highest risk is with African American males, then we must address the nuances (psychological, cultural, and religious) of this social relationship, which includes social behaviors and our individual thoughts about it, that lead us away from safe sexual encounters.

Intervention and Trauma

There have been a few attempts to address the gap in effective HIV prevention and intervention efforts for African American women. DiClemente and Wingood (1995) proposed and implemented a Social Skills Training intervention for African American women based on social cognitive theory and theories of gender and power. This training included ethnic pride, personal responsibility for decision making, sexual assertiveness and communication training, condom use, and cognitive coping skills. But further interventions that acknowledge that there is a need for specific interventions to address culture and mind-sets have not been developed. I believe that intervention strategies that are directed to the unique needs of African American women are few and almost nonexistent because of mental health profession's reluctance to accept the direct influence of racioethnicity and racial trauma.

Most interventions for African American women have only addressed the theoretical perspectives in the mental health field. They have either attempted to make the client fit the intervention (safe sex) or stretch the intervention to fit the client (behavioral change strategies). The statistical numbers regarding African American women underscore the fact that this approach is not working. Jackson (2000) makes the case that in order to work with this population, mental health professionals need to identify the differences among certain variables and how they interact. The specific variables are intrapsychic, cultural, and social constructions. All of these areas impact the behaviors of African American women and leave them vulnerable to contracting HIV/AIDS.

There are some specific variables that impact the social and psychological health of African American women and their ability to cope in this society. These areas are the historical legacy of slavery, racism, sexual assault, devalued self-image, and stereotyping (Jackson, 2000). Psychological trauma is at the core of each one of these unique experiences of African American women that are often overlooked. Jackson states that not all African American women have been traumatized, but there is evidence that a significant number have or will be affected on one or more of these dimensions yet will remain silent. Please note that psychological trauma is an intrapsychic issue, and racial trauma is not included in the psychological literature that addresses trauma. Jackson asserts that racial trauma's absence in the psychological trauma literature is a way that mental health theorists continue to deny its existence.

Gardere (2002) asserts that there is a link between many of the destructive patterns of African Americans and the trauma of slavery and racism in this country. He defines it as Post Traumatic Slavery Disorder (PTSD), a psychiatric disorder that fits the description of the DSM-IV's Post-Traumatic Stress Disorder, but is specific to the residuals of slavery and institutionalized racism. Gardere asserts that the damage caused by the extreme and long-lasting injury of slavery is pervasive, long-lasting, and has affected virtually every person of color whose history was blighted by slavery and colonialism (p. 27). Unfortunately, the prevailing attitude in the United States is that African Americans should get over the slavery issue and the long-term racism. This attitude denies that there is any residual mental trauma experienced by the persons confronted with racism, who are still the most discriminated against group in this country.

I contend that there are variables, often overlooked by mental health professionals, that have had and still have an impact on African American women's lives. The result is the lack of coping skills and dysfunctional behavioral patterns that influence their ability to choose health-promoting and life-empowering behaviors. Richardson and Wade (1999) concur with this perspective and assert that African American women's struggle to hold on to a sense of dignity in a hostile environment has resulted in maladaptive patterns of thinking, believing, and acting that is often misunderstood. They identify seven emotional inherited beliefs that need to be addressed in a supportive and therapeutic way (pp. 22–24):

1. There will never be enough of anything I need, especially love.
2. I'm not good enough to be loved.
3. I'll lose anyone who gets close to me.
4. It's not safe for me to face my anger.
5. No matter what I do, it won't make a difference.
6. I have to control everyone and everything around me to protect myself from being hurt again.
7. My body is not my own.

These beliefs are similar to areas that are addressed in cognitive behavioral therapies, that assert that what we think and believe precede our behavior. Jackson and Greene (2000) believe that psychodynamic theories and their techniques can be helpful because they provide tools to help African American women to explore the relationship between historical emotional learning and their emotional defensive responses of their experiences.

Cultural Influences

We must not downplay or minimize the influence of cultural and/or religious influences to our behaviors or allow others to continue to do so. Because culture is complex and not easy to define, and even more complex is the relationship between race and culture, such influence is often overlooked in research and intervention strategies. Jackson (2000) concurs that culture continues to be misunderstood and misapplied to various groups. Culture does influence behavior. The notion of what is meant by culture, how it influences one's view of health, and what would be considered a useful intervention is an appropriate start (Jackson, 2000, p. 6).

Bagley and Carroll (1998) assert that African Americans, in terms of their mental health, must be understood in their social context because they have to contend with pressures due to the burdens of racism and oppression. The mental health profession has not always been open to the African American clients and African Americans have not trusted the profession. Consequently, because race has always significantly impacted their lives, African Americans have instituted their own indigenous support systems (Bagley & Carroll, 1998). All of these indigenous support systems hinge on the African American family and include the extended family, church, organizations, values, and internal and external coping strategies.

Boyd-Franklin (1989) asserts a multisystems approach for African Americans families in therapy. Her multisystems levels begin with the individual and spiral out to subsystems of the family household, extended family, non-blood kin and friends, church and community resources, and social service agencies and other outside systems. She asserts that because African Americans are new to therapy, an individual may describe an intrapsychic or interpersonal issue, when in fact it is a family therapy issue. Consequently, this multilevel system can work for the individual as well as the family.

This concept of multilevel approach to supporting the African American person that is based in the family support is important to any and all interventions for African American women. Just the infusion of racio-ethnic pride is not enough; there must also be interventions that draw support that is consistent with the cultural norms of the African American community.

Dana (1998) believes there are distinct reasons why cultural competence is not infused in psychological assessments and interventions. He believes there are attitudinal and technical limitations, which include: worldview and cultural or racial identities; acculturation; bias in the form or racism; ethnocentrism and ethnorelativism; research beliefs and practices; and Anglo American standards for service delivery, assessment instruments, diagnosis, interventions, and training.

Cultural competency is defined as acquiring the attitudes, knowledge, and skills needed to function effectively in a pluralistic democratic society and to interact, negotiate, and communicate with peoples from diverse backgrounds. Cultural competency fosters and expands a person's ability to interact effectively with persons from diverse backgrounds and persons who have diverse ways of doing things. The relationship of these three variables should be integrated into any training curriculums developed for African Americans women about HIV/AIDS. But this cultural competency must integrate the multiple layers and interactive effects of culture in the lives of African American women, and not minimize it to behavioral measures. We must see the behavioral outcomes— effective and consistent condom use as an outgrowth of a health promotion consciousness. In turn, the consciousness comes from a healthy social psychological attitude that includes overcoming any and all traumatic issues (racial and sexual), and healthy attitudes about the self in relationship to this society, the culture, and relationships with significant others.

Behavioral Change

Last, but certainly not the least, is the outcome problem of behavioral change. How do we encourage African American women to move from risky behaviors to safe sex behavior? Do we stop focusing on behavioral change and just look at the social psychological and cultural underpinnings of the problem? I would think not! But I believe that once we address these underlying issues, we must not limit our strategies to only one model of behavior change. We must become eclectic in our approach and find interventions that fit the complexity of the problem at hand.

DiClemente and Wingood (1995) assert that current models of behavior change have provided useful guidance for understanding HIV risk-reduction practices, but these models have failed to consider a host of contextual social factors that shape the reality of risk and potential risk-reduction for African American women. We must stop minimizing the sociocultural factors (socio-economic, sociocultural, psychosocial, sociopolitical, moral, and spiritual) and assess the "real" factors that lead to the escalating levels of infection in the African American community, and especially in women. The plain truth is that most of the interventions to arrest the disease in African American communities and accessible to African Americans tend to mirror strategies that were used for predominantly white and gay communities. The prevailing HIV/AIDS outreach activities that still utilize strategies developed for white gay males do not and have not impacted the HIV/AIDS epidemic in the African American community. In addition, interventions that focus just on African American women are very few in number. Evidently, interventions that are not founded on quality research and insight into the true nature of the target population, and instead only replicate interventions for Euro-Americans, will not help us to retard the spread of the disease.

A case in point is the use of only one stage of change behavioral model. The Transtheoretical Change Model (Prochaska et al., 1992) was designed to describe the stages of change people go through when changing behaviors and is the predominant theory used in HIV prevention and intervention activities. These stages are: Precontemplation, Contemplation, Preparation, Action, and Maintenance.

There are more than one stage of change behavioral model and possibly one that is more suitable to the complex needs of African American women. Crosby et al. (2002) asserts that the precaution adoption process model directly targets the problem with African American women in a rural setting who were unengaged by the potential threat of HIV infection. I think this state of being unengaged is also rampant in urban areas and across social class in the African American community.

The precaution adoption process model (PAPM) identifies seven stages in a process that moves a person to adopt a precaution (Weinstein, 1988; Weinstein & Sandman, 1992). Their seven stages are: unaware of issue, unengaged by the issue, deciding about acting, decided not to act, decided to act, acting, and maintenance. I like the expansion of the stages because a person could be made aware yet remain unengaged by the issue. This stage of being unengaged can be the place where African American women allow their culture, religion, gender roles, and other factors to block moving them to the place of decision making. Prevention and intervention activities need to go beyond information to the type of strategies that will help them engage and recognize that they are at risk.

In this stage of change process, only engagement will bring the woman to a place of decision. But the other good feature is that there are three stages of decision making: deciding about acting, decided not to act, and decided to act. This model does not assume that decision making is a straightforward activity and that it always leads to the right decision. I believe this is the place where the intervention must include the monitoring, mentoring, support, and encouragement that can be given through multilevel systems in the African American community. The intervention must be designed to meet the cultural and relational needs of women.

African American women become more involved when there is an atmosphere of true trust and concern. If they are already mistrustful of the health and social service agencies in this country, then interventions that encourage trust and support are mandatory. In addition, to help a person make a decision about behaviors in their private, sexual lives there needs to be a supportive, "sister-to-sister" environment. A stage of change model that allows for the multiple and complex factors that influence behavior change for African American women, as well as, leaves room for the infusion of sociocultural as well as mentoring relationships could be crucial to interventions that effectively help African American women.

In addition, the interventions for African American women must see cultural consciousness beyond race and ethnic pride, to a social cognitive confrontation of race, religion, and gender issues that influence the choices that African American women make. Along with the confrontation and deconstruction of myths and beliefs, there need to be tools, role-plays, and role models and mentors that can assist women on relational level—not just didactic interventions.

Final Thoughts

Tina Turner made a phrase famous after confronting years of emotional and physical abuse and trauma: "What's love got to do with it?" I believe that loving yourself has everything to do with it. When it all boils down to what mind-set will really lead African American women to behavioral change, it will come back to interventions that lead us to self-esteem, self-efficacy, and loving ourselves. These interventions will save our lives. This is not only plain talk, but also the plain truth that can lead us to positive and effective actions.

REFERENCES

Azibo, D. A. 1996. "Personality, Clinical, and Social Psychological Research on Blacks: Appropriate and Inappropriate Research Frameworks." In D. A. Azibo (Ed.), *African Psychology in Historial Perspective and Related Commentary* (pp. 203–34). Trenton, NJ: Africa World Press.

Bagley, C. A., and J. Carroll. 1998. "Healing Forces in African American Families." In H. I. McCubbin, E. A. Thompson, A. I. Thompson, and J. A. Futtrell (Eds.), *Resiliency in African-American Families* (pp. 117–42). Thousand Oaks, CA: Sage Publications.

Belgrave, F. Z. 1992. "Improving Health Outcomes of African Americans: A Challenge for African American Psychologists." In A.K.H. Burlew, W. C. Banks, H. P. McAdoo, and D. A. Azibo (Eds.), *African American Psychology: Theory, Research, and Practice* (pp. 356–58). Newbury Park, CA: Sage.

Betsch Cole, J., and B. Guy-Sheftall. 2003. *Gender Talk: The Struggle for Women's Equality in African American Communities.* New York: One World, Ballantine Books.

Bowleg, L., F. Z. Belgrave, and C. A. Reisen. 2000. "Gender Roles, Power Strategies and Precautionary Sexual Self-Efficacy: Implications for Black and Latina Women's HIV/AIDS Protection Behaviors." *Sex Roles* 42(7–8):613–35.

Boyd-Franklin, N. 1989. *Black Families in Therapy: A Multisystems Approach.* New York: Guilford Press.

Bradford, J., and D. Kennamer. 1995. *"HIV-Related Knowledge, Attitudes and Behavior of Virginians: 1995 African-American Sample. A Study Conducted by the Virginia HIV Prevention Community Planning Committee."* Virginia Commonwealth University.

Crosby, R. A., W. L. Yarber, R. J. DiClemente, G. M. Wingood, and B. Meyerson. 2002. "HIV-Associated Histories, Perceptions, and Practices among Low-income African American Women: Does Rural Residence Matter?" *American Journal of Public Health,* 92(4):655–59.

Dana, R. H. 1998. *Understanding Cultural Identity in Intervention and Assessment.* Thousand Oaks, CA: Sage Publications.

DiClemente, R. J. Fall, 1992. "African Americans and AIDS: Confronting the Challenge of AIDS in the African-American Community." *Ethnicity and Disease* 2, 358–360.

DiClemente, R. J., and G. M. Wingood. 1995. "A Randomized Controlled Trial of an HIV Sexual Risk-Reduction Intervention for Young African American Women." *Journal of the American Medical Association,* 16(2–4):1271–76.

Fullilove, M. T., R. Fullilove, K. Haynes, and W. Gross. 1990. "Black Women and AIDS Prevention: A View towards Understanding the Gender Rules." *Journal of Sex Research* 27, 47–64.

Gardere, Jeffrey. 2002. *Love Prescription: Ending the War between Black Men and Women.* New York: Kensington Publishing Group.

Gergen, K. J. 2001. *Social Construction in Context.* Thousand Oaks, CA: Sage Publications.

Hearn, K. D., and L. R. Jackson. 2002. "African American Women and HIV Risk: Exploring the Effects of Gender and Social Dynamics on Behavior." *African American Research Perspectives* 8(1):163–73.

Jackson, L. C. 2000. "The New Multiculturalism and Psychodynamic Theory: Psychodynamic Psychotherapy and African American women." In L. C. Jackson and B. Greene (Eds.). *Psychotherapy with African American Women: Innovations in Psychodynamic Perspectives and Practice* (pp. 1–14). New York: Guilford Press.

Jackson, L. C., and Greene, B. (Eds.). 2000. *Psychotherapy with African American Women: Innovations in Psychodynamic Perspectives and Practice.* New York: Guilford Press.

Johnson, E. H., L. A. Jackson, et al. 1994. "What Is the Significance of Black-White Differences in Risky Sexual Behavior?" *Journal of the National Medical Association* 86(10):745–59. Morehouse School of Medicine, Department of Family Medicine, Atlanta, GA.

Jones, C., and K. Shorter-Gooden. 2003. *Shifting: The Double Lives of Black Women in America.* New York: HarperCollins Publishers.

Kimberly, J. A., and J. M. Serovich. 1999. *The Role of Family and Friend Social Support in Reducing Risk Behaviors among HIV Positive Gay Men.* New York: Guilford Publishing.

Kline, A., E. Kline, and E. Oken. 1992. "Minority Women and Sexual Choice in the Age of AIDS." *Social Science and Medicine* 34, 447–57.

Lester, B. Fall. 1993. "The Social Context of HIV Transmission in the African-American Community." *Ethnicity and Disease* 3(4):387–94.

McCubbin, H. I., E. A. Thompson, A. I. Thompson, and J. A. Futrell (Eds.). 1998. *Resiliency in African-American Families.* Thousand Oaks, CA: Sage Publications.

McNair, L. D., and C. M. Prather. 2004. "African American Women and AIDS: Factors Influencing Risk and Reaction to HIV Disease." *Journal of Black Psychology* 30(1):106–23.

McNair, L. D., and G. W. Roberts. 1997. "Pervasive and Persistent Risks: Factors Influencing African American Women's HIV/AIDS Vulnerability." *Journal of Black Psychology* 23(2):180–91.

Miller, L. C., D. M. Burns, and S. Rothspan. 1995. "The Dynamics of African-American Relationships." In P. Kalbfleish and M. Cody (Eds.), *Gender, Power and Communication in Human Relationships* (pp. 163–88). Hillside, NJ: Lawrence Erlbaum Associates.

Overby, K. J., and S. M. Kegeles. 1994. "The Impact of AIDS on an Urban Population of High-risk Female Minority Adolescents: Implications for Intervention." *Journal of Adolescent Health* 15, 216–27.

Peeler, L. E. 2002. *Sex, Lies and Social Constructions: HIV-Related Knowledge, Attitudes and Behaviors of African-Americans in Buffalo, New York—2000 Sample.* Buffalo, NY: Prominent Life Resources.

Prochaska, J. O., C. C. DiClemente, and J. C. Norcross. 1992. "In Search of How People Change: Applications to Addictive Behaviors." *American Psychologist* 47, 1102–14.

Richardson, B. I., and B. Wade. 1999. *What Mama Couldn't Tell Us about Love.* New York: HarperCollins.

Taylor, B. M. 1995. "Gender-Power Relationships and Safer Sex Negotiation." *Journal of Advanced Nursing* 22, 687–93.

Weinstein, N. D. 1988. "The Precaution Adoption Process." *Health Psychology* 7, 355–86.

Weinstein, N. D., A. J. Rothman, and S. R. Sutton. 1998. "Stage Theories of Health Behavior: Conceptual and Methodological Issues." *Health Psychology* 17(3):290–99.

Weinstein, N. D., and P. Sandman. 2002. "The Precaution Adoption Process Model and Its Application." In R. J. DiClemente, R. A. Crosby, and M. C. Kegler (Eds.), *Emerging Theories in Health Promotion and Practice and Research.* New York: Jossey-Bass/Wiley.

Williams, P. B., O. Keundayo, and I. E. Udezulu. 2003. "An Ethnically Sensitive and Gender-Specific HIV/AIDS Assessment of African American Women: A Comparative Study of Urban and Rural American Communities." *Family Community Health* 26(2):108–24.

Wingood, G. M., and R. J. DiClemente. 1997. "Consequences of Having a Physically Abusive Partner on the Condom Use and Sexual Negotiation Practices of Young Adult African-American Women." *American Journal of Public Health* 87, 1016–18.

———. 1998. "Pattern Influences and Gender Related Factors Associated with Noncondom Use Among Young Adult African American Women." *American Journal of Community Psychology* 26, 29–49.

Wingood, G. M., R. J. DiClemente, D. H. McCree, K. Harrington, and S. L. Davies. 2001. "Dating Violence and the Sexual Health of Black Adolescent Females." *Pediatrics* 107(5):72. Available online at http://pediatrics.aappublications.org/cgi/content/full/107/5/e72.

Wingood, G. M., D. Hunter-Gamble, and R. J. DiClemente. 1993. "A Pilot Study of Sexual Communication and Negotiation among Young African American Women: Implications for HIV Prevention." *Journal of Black Psychology* 19, 190–203.

8

Allowing Illness in Order to Heal: Sojourning the African American Woman and the AIDS Pandemic

RENEE BOWMAN DANIELS

The AIDS pandemic presents one of the most unique medical and social dilemmas of our time. This is especially true for African American women who are suffering from the silence of AIDS and dying in the shadows. Imagine, in the United States, in 2001, HIV/AIDS was the leading cause of death for African American women ages 25–34, and we comprised 67 percent of the female population diagnosed with AIDS in 2003. How reflective this is of the cultural and historical struggle that has enslaved a community for centuries, as we have allowed ourselves to be postured as pillars of strength, healers, and caretakers for everyone but ourselves. As a result of adopting an edifice of strength based on the denial of our own illness, we now suffer the consequences, which endanger the very goal we sought to achieve, the continuation of the people. This chapter will examine, from an Africentric perspective, the sociocultural factors which surround the pandemic of HIV/AIDS among African American women. The chapter presents the concept of empowerment for wellness for the collective survival of the African American woman and the community in which she is a centerpiece. Recommendations and strategies are profiled that will "allow illness in order to heal."

HIV/AIDS is killing us. Our community, our women, our men, our children, our families, our future—all lie under siege to a tragedy happening in silence. It is estimated that 39 million people are living with HIV/AIDS worldwide. HIV/AIDS, cast as the health catastrophe of our lifetime, was originally characterized as an epidemic of gender (male) and sexual orientation (homosexual). Women were an afterthought early in the HIV/AIDS epidemic. Today, however, there is a woman's face on this pandemic. We are accepting our fair share of the disease, as evidenced by the fact that 27 percent of the AIDS cases diagnosed in 2003 were women. Women of color, and in particular African American women, are disproportionately affected by HIV/AIDS. What accounts for this disparity, especially when the review of some of the demographics suggest an improving picture of African American life? African Americans make up 12.9 percent of the U.S. population, and there are those who predict a reclaiming of the second largest group category in the U.S census by the year 2010, consisting of African Americans, Hispanics, Asian Americans, and Native Americans (AHANA). We are a young population, with a median age of 29.5 years, in comparison with 35.3 years for the total U.S. population.

Our educational attainment has improved: 72 percent of African Americans over the age of 25 have at least a high school diploma (in the 1990 census the figure was 63 percent), and 14 percent have a bachelor's degree or higher (as compared to 11 percent in 1990). The median income for African Americans households is $29,470, and 46 percent of all African American householders own their own home (African American Legends, n.d., p. 1). While these statistical compilations are encouraging, there is still one fact that remains; disparity in African American life remains steadfast. Our community bears the burden of inequitable poverty, crime, imprisonment, and unemployment. Even more unsettling are the racial and ethnic disparities in health. In fact, the overall health status of African Americans is alarming. The National Center for Health Statistics (NCHS) reports that African Americans are far more likely to be assessed in only fair or poor health than any other racial group, and the rate of disease among African Americans is almost double the rate of other races. African Americans are generally 1.5 times as likely to be sick and die as Caucasians (Avery, 1992, p. 36; Department of Health and Human Services, 1985).

In the last three years of the 1980s, public health officials reported increases among African Americans in diseases that had been steadily declining since the beginning of the century, and considered on the verge of eradication less than a decade ago. These diseases include tuberculosis, hepatitis A, measles, mumps, and whooping cough complicated by ear infections. The *Healthy People 2000* report published by the Office of Minority Health states that the leading causes of death among African American men and women continue to be heart disease, cancer, stroke, lung disease, pneumonia, diabetes, and injuries. And then there is the HIV/AIDS pandemic, which since its beginning has affected the minority population in a majority way. Something is amiss with this twenty-first-century picture.

JUST THE HIV/AIDS FACTS

Globally, the picture of HIV/AIDS is hard to believe. Entire nations have felt the rampage. During 2004 it is estimated that 4.9 million people became newly infected with HIV, including 640,000 children under the age of 15. Moreover, 3.1 million people died of AIDS in 2004, and children accounted for over half a million of these deaths. The saddest report of all is that most people living with HIV are unaware that they are infected (UNAIDS, 2004). In the United States, the overall number of AIDS cases diagnosed in 2003 (43,171) increased 4.6 percent over the number diagnosed in 2002. As the epidemic ages, new at-risk groups have taken the stage, including racial and ethnic (AHANA) communities, women, and adolescents. In 1992, women with AIDS accounted for only 14 percent of adults and adolescents living with AIDS. By the end of 2003, this percentage grew to 22 percent. The annual number of AIDS diagnoses has increased 15 percent among women, in comparison to 1 percent among men. Women represented 27 percent (11,498) of the 43,171 AIDS cases diagnosed in 2003. Caring the burden of this increase are African American women and children. In fact in 2003, African Americans accounted for 49 percent of the newly diagnosed cases, with a case rate per 100,000 of 9.5 times that of Caucasians. The rate of AIDS diagnoses for African American women (50.2/100,000) was 25 times the rate for Caucasian women (2.0/100,000) (CDC, 2003). Although African American women are only 13 percent of the female population in the United States, we represent the majority of new AIDS cases among women, accounting for 67 percent of the estimated female AIDS cases in 2003 (CDC, 2004). HIV was the leading cause of death for African American women ages 25–34 in 2001, compared to the sixth leading cause for women in general in the United States (NCHS, 2003). HIV/AIDS is truly a major health crisis for African Americans, and in particular the African American woman.

At the end of the twentieth century it was predicted that heterosexual contact would become the primary means of spreading HIV infection in most industrialized countries over the next several decades. As of 2003, heterosexual contact with an infected partner or a man at high risk for HIV infection accounted for 80 percent of HIV infections in women. "Statistics indicate that the most frequent mode of transmission of the HIV virus to African-American women is through sexual contact with African American men who were intravenous drug users and/or gay, or bisexual" (Richie, 1994, p. 184). African American women are also becoming infected at younger ages than their ethnic and racial counterparts. Compounding this is a mean survival time for African Americans once diagnosed with acquired immunodeficiency syndrome of 8 months, compared to 18–24 months for Caucasians (CDC, 1995).

Since 1981, when the first case of a woman with AIDS was reported in the United States, limited attention has been directed to clinical practice, research, or public discussion of women and the HIV/AIDS epidemic. The first National Conference on Women and HIV infection, held in December 1990 and sponsored by the Public Health Service (PHS), found that little was known about women and AIDS. What is known is that HIV-infected women acknowledge more psychological and physical abuse than noninfected women. Life in general for many African American women is a series of interpersonal transactions that cause tremendous amounts of distress. A survey conducted by the National Health and Nutrition Examination Surveys (NHANES) found that over half of the African American women participants between the ages of 18 and 25 reported living in a state of psychological distress (Avery, 1992). Exactly what is meant by distress? The American Heritage dictionary defines distress as "causing strain, anxiety or suffering . . . a condition of being in need of immediate assistance" (p. 541). In search of further clarification of this condition, the California Black Women's Health Project conducted a study of 1,300 African American women. Findings included African American women feeling "overwhelmed by the pursuit of perfectionism, mediating family conflicts, and challenging the criticisms and doubts of others" (Curphey, 2003, p. 3). Now, add to this our new center stage in the pandemic of AIDS.

To understand the phenomena of the African American woman suffering and dying in the shadows of a worldwide pandemic, our community must begin to understand the plight of the African American women's cultural and historical legacy, the disempowering concept of illness as it is perceived in our community and family structures, and the successes of our struggles in this land we call our home. It is only then that we will be empowered to act expeditiously to heal and embrace a healthy community.

LIVING AND DYING IN THE SHADOWS

The health status of African American women reflects the historical and environmental structures of the pre–Civil War era (Lawson & Thompson, 1994). It has been 142 years since the Emancipation Proclamation became effective, yet African American women are still held in bondage. For so long our strength, love, and determination have been focused on the welfare of our community. We have been taught to reorder our own priorities and to find enrichment through our commitment to the welfare of others. We are the wives, partners, daughters, sisters, and mothers of a community plagued by illness and the pandemic of AIDS, but we ourselves are also losing the AIDS battle (Sharp, 1993).

African American women share a cultural and historical legacy that not only provides African heritage, but also encompasses a life of exploitation and oppression through colonization, enslavement, codified apartheid, de facto segregation, or other expressions of individual and institutional racism. In a world that is dominated by "isms" such as racism and sexism, the African American female suffers from her status of being Black and female. This is further compounded if she is a single parent in a society where the two-parent family is perceived to be the "norm."

To be part of the African American, Black, Afro-American, Negro, or Coloured community means a yoking to racist stereotypes that associate our communities with criminal or deviant behavior. Much of the salient social science literature, written by others about our African American community, proliferates the European American myth about our lack of morality and our hypersexuality. Utilizing race as the relevant label of identification, Black people are seen on a positive domain only in terms of good "ball" players, musicians, dancers, rhythm and blues and jazz singers, jokesters, and unskilled laborers; in other words, as servants to the majority culture. And what of the African American female's image of herself and her life?

Historically, sexism has played a major role in robbing us of our self-esteem and devaluing our femaleness. Pre–Civil War bondage found African American women treated as organic property, denied the right to their virginity, and cast in the role of breeder and sex object, ready for use at anyone's leisure. Post–Civil War bondage placed African American women in a unique juxtaposition of prostitution and prostration. Medical care was provided because we were economic assets. However, the medical care and practice was predicated on physiological differences, rooted in a racist ideology that believed in the genetic inferiority of black women.

Today, African American women continue to find definition in the context of human relationships. Through these relationships we take on the role of nurturer, shoulder the burden of caretaker and caregiver, and affix ourselves as helpmate. In exchange we are celebrated for our unique devotion to the task of mothering, our innate ability to bear tremendous burdens, and for our ever-increasing availability as sex objects (Hooks, 1981). Now let us add to this the myth of the Black matriarch. This theory casts African American women as both dominating and castrating. The matriarch is idealized for her strength, liberated attitude, assertiveness, and self-sufficiency. As the matriarch she is responsible for the survival of the family and the community, while within the same breath, she is blamed for the so called disintegration of the African American family (Staples, 1994).

Make no mistake, this divisive theory espoused by social scientists really only serves to emasculate our men and our community, and provide the impetus for the African American women's sojourn into a life of self-denial and self-blame. Seen as this monument of strength, the African American women is left with little room to be ill or have any problems, engage in help-seeking behaviors, or utilize resources.

We do not allow ourselves to be ill. Many have recognized this cultural and societal dynamic in the African American community. It allows us to distance ourselves from illness and the pandemic of AIDS, which in many ways is like every other health, social, and economic crisis that African Americans have faced for generations. Our impulse to distance ourselves from HIV/AIDS is less a response to the disease than a reaction to the myriad of social issues that surround the disease and give it meaning (Dalton, 1989). African Americans have been and continue to be blamed for the origin and spread of AIDS. After all it has been suggested that HIV/AIDS originated with Africans, and because of their sexual prowess, they contributed significantly to the spread of the virus/disease.

Compound a deep-seated suspicion and mistrust for a health system that recognizes African Americans as subjects of programs to reduce fertility and demonstrate the effects of untreated disease, and I would say the denial and rejection of the illness is a buffer between a hostile environment and the community. Several studies (Braithwaite & Taylor, 2001; Williams et al., 2003) document the ever-present negative attitudes and feelings, the lack of trust, and the misconceptions held by the African American community in reference to HIV/AIDS. In fact Williams et al. indicates one of the most surprising aspects of their study was the association of the current epidemic with a "government genocidal" plot against the African American race.

Illness is not a welcomed concept in the African American community. One speaks more of being "sick," for this is tolerated although not acceptable. Illness is an experience, a complex set of ways in which the sick person, the members of the family, and other social networks understand, live with, and respond to the symptoms and disability (Kleinman, 1988). Being ill is disruptive and disordering because it impinges on our sense of who we are and our important social relationships. HIV/AIDS, although fitting the definition of a disease ("a biophysical condition") is also an illness. As an illness it is often experienced as overwhelming, unpredictable, and uncontrollable because it paralyzes the person's ability to manage life, to plan, and to act.

The human response to illness is to give it meaning, to interpret it, to reorder the disordering experience. To make sense of what is happening to us, we draw upon socially available categories from a large cultural repertoire and from personal and family stories and meanings absorbed from our particular ethnic and religious backgrounds. In the case of minor illnesses, the interpretations might include our underlying definitions of health and illness, and our notions about why we get sick and how to get well. Seriously disruptive illnesses are likely to evoke further interpretations about the meaning of life, moral responsibility, suffering, relationships, and death. (Freund & McGuire, 1991, p. 157)

AIDS in the general population was historically interpreted as the "gay" disease, followed by the conclusion that this is "God's way of ridding the earth of undesirables," under which category the community places intravenous (IV) drug users. Under what category should we place the African American woman and her child? How does the community come to understand that a woman is now sick, and dying because she perhaps loved another, whose history or present lifestyle includes drug abuse, needle sharing, or a bisexual, homosexual relationship? Can we be strong enough to acknowledge an illness that is robbing the community of its childbearing force? Can we admit that the African American woman, who has been the centerpiece in the struggle for equality, dignity, and honor and contributed to every scene of the African American drama (Ashante & Mattison, 1991), might have to step down from her role as caregiver and became an earthly vessel needing care? And are we as a community ready to truly understand the relationship between love and sexuality and the African American women's role, position, and status in intimate relationships? This understanding is necessary to begin to undo the "blackface" of AIDS.

Sexual relationships between men and women have often been identified by the female gender in terms of obligations; it was the woman's duty. However, the social dynamics of the African American woman's sexual experience placed her in the position of being seen as excessively sexual and promiscuous. As mainstream culture promoted repressive attitudes towards sexuality, rooted in group values systems and practices manipulated by racism and sexism, the African American community banished the extremely subjective and stigmatized experience of sexuality to a position of silence. Therefore, African American women are cautious and have limited experience with acknowledging or sharing with one another or their mate the interconnections of our emotional, sexual, and reproductive experiences. In essence, we have become disempowered through own historical and contemporary experiences, and cannot allow or acknowledge illness, particularly those emanating from our sexual experiences.

ALLOWING ILLNESS IN ORDER TO HEAL

Our community is under attack by what has been identified as the health catastrophe of our lifetime, AIDS. It has a divide and conquer strategy, which is not new to the African American community. However, as we continue to struggle for life, progress is often threatened by a weakening of our social and personal resolve (Billingsley, 1992). Despite these situations and daily experiences that continue to oppress our community, we remain an unconquered people whose strength is found in our interdependence, collectiveness, and our sense of peoplehood. We must remember, though, to be unconquered is not synonymous with fairing well. As Dalton (1989, p. 219) points out, "we have been so busy expressing our fears that we have failed to express our hopes." We must draw strength and advantage from the situations that oppress us because that substantial gains and progress in our community in the past.

The concept of empowerment for well-being must be reenergized in the African American community. The African American women must redefine her status and reclaim the importance of self. She must remember that it is through her visions and dreams that our people have been kept alive. Now, in the midst of this pandemic, the African American women finds herself once again struggling for her survival and the survival of our people will require a refocus, a readjustment, creative health promotions, and lifesaving program initiatives.

But how do African American women in particular begin the process of empowerment, which must be thoroughly integrated into everyday life experiences and situations? How do feelings of powerlessness translate into action or inaction on African American women's health issues? How does a person, long denied, begin to believe she has a right to allow illness in order to heal (Avery, 1992)?

REFOCUS, READJUSTMENT, AND ATTITUDINAL CHANGE

Treatment of all women relative to HIV/AIDS will be more effective if it is based on an understanding of the societal context in which women live as well as their relational needs. The community must perceive and understand the consequences of a disempowered state within which African American women quietly live, as well as other life issues that contribute to their inability to protect herself from infection. These include psychosocial, cultural, and legal barriers to her decision making; the lack of economic alternatives, with the consequent dependence on a man for support; the societal role of women as primary caretakers of children, husbands, and parents; the well-known case of women's lower literacy in some countries, as well as their limited mobility and limited access to information; and let us not forget societal attitudes about sexuality (Williams, 1991). Health promotion and prevention efforts have, to a great extent, centered on educating women about "safe sex," but advising women to use condoms truly reflects a lack of knowledge about gender role and power issues within the African American community. Our efforts must demonstrate an understanding of the risk factors so prevalent in the African American community.

Lack of insurance, inadequate medical attention, and general poor health do contribute directly to increased infection rates among African American women. But what about the phenomenon of a criminal justice system in which people of color are disproportionately incarcerated? In the U.S. prison system there are three times as many AIDS cases as in the general U.S. population. Subsequently, the increase in the number of African American ex-offenders living with HIV/AIDS corresponds with the increasing infection rates for African American women who for the most part contract HIV through heterosexual relationships (Browne-Marshall, 2004).

Additionally, many women are either unaware of or maintain a certain naiveté in reference to their male partners' risks for HIV infection. These risks include unprotected sex with multiple partners, partners living on the "down-low," bisexuality, or IV drug use. African American women must be able to see themselves in any proposed preventive service models, and to see myself I must understand how this program will benefit my children, my companions, and my community.

African American women are more likely to become sensitized to AIDS issues, to engage in empowering behavior such as HIV testing, to encourage prophylactic use, and to have an enhanced perception of HIV risk if the messages stress culturally relevant values. Such values include linking behavior change to pride in one's culture, noting the adverse effect of AIDS in African American communities, and stressing family responsibility to protect the children (Land, 1994; Kalichman et al., 1992). Prevention efforts should focus on those methods that women can control, such as the use of spermicides and physical barrier methods of protection that also serve as contraception. Additionally, service providers must refocus prevention efforts on educating our men and include grassroots community involvement that will encourage men to talk with one another about their sexual behavior (Avery, 1992). This is particularly important considering the down-low experience, which describes men who deny they are homosexual but secretly have sex with other men while maintaining heterosexual relationships. Thus, a new element has been added to at-risk behaviors, and prevention efforts must include this new twist. When we can stop punishing our women, our men, and our children for their behavior and provide lifesaving information in an atmosphere of trust, perhaps the community attitude about HIV/AIDS will change. Remember, for the most part the African American community is still very conservative.

Our community is long overdue for an attitude adjustment which will serve as the precursor to behavioral change. We must change our attitude about ourselves. No longer do we have the time or the circumstance in which we can allow others to usurp, manipulate, exalt, degrade, alter, exploit, suppress, or turn back against African American women, our image of self and of our community. "We must stop loving our sons and raising our daughters and give both the love needed for responsible self-respect" (Avery, 1992, p. 37).

Perhaps then the African American woman and man will develop the atmosphere in which conversations can occur regarding those issues that impact on the health of the community, such as a roof over our heads, a meal on the table, dignity and self-worth, quality health care, the education of our children, economic stability, self-determination, and sexual intimacies and behaviors and their consequences.

We must understand that the stereotypes about our moral character and hypersexuality are convenient racist and sexist labels. These labels foster a socialization process that pits us against our men and holds the community hostage by way of mental enslavement to the concept of deviance and the recurrent fear of further stigmatization. The African American community must learn that labels dictate process and must empower itself community to accept the illness. In order to heal, we must engage in a dissociative relationship with current labels and classifications. Our messages, our literature, the physical environments of our programs, and communities must focus on old terms that have more acceptable meanings and circumstances. Instead of using the words *sick* or *ill*, we need to promote the concept of healthy and unhealthy communities, families, men, women, and children. This concept is without stigma yet personal enough so one can link health to the welfare of the community. We must organize around the promotion of a healthy community focusing on those facts and actions that inform and educate rather than blame and victimize. In the African Americans community, we believe in "calling a spade and spade," so we should tell the HIV/AIDS messages like it is, in a language without labels.

The African American community is unhealthy at the present because there is a condition one can acquire that will stop the body's immune system from protecting it from all the different viruses, infections, and diseases that are in our environment. The future of our community is being jeopardized by a condition called acquired immunodeficiency syndrome.

The use of this language first teaches by actually describing the condition. The use of the actual medical term promotes the demystification, lessens the stigmatization, and removes the label of deviance from this "illness." The African American community accepts conditions, as typified by the terms *high blood pressure* versus *hypertension*, *sugar* versus *diabetes*. It is all a matter of words and their symbolism.

TEACHING A COMMUNITY OLD TRICKS

There has always been, and continues to be, tremendous strength in the African American community. Perhaps it is time to ask ourselves: how have we survived? As directions and path are forged at this most significant crossroads, let us not forget to investigate and then celebrate the remarkable successes that so many women and families have experienced, and learn from these in order to progress in the face of ever-more pressing obstacles. To build a healthy community, service providers, whether indigenous or outside professionals, must utilize a holistic approach, a comprehensive systems treatment approach that views the family as a whole, focuses on relationship building, and demonstrates care for the African American women in all her roles. Our African American community must implement and then evaluate community interventions that will prevent further transmission of AIDS, and specifically target women who are at high risk.

Educational outreach and condom distribution, as well as teaching drug addicts how to clean their needles or offering a free "needle exchange" program, have proved effective in reducing the rate of HIV transmission. This type of intervention has proved effective in Zaire, where prostitutes were given condoms and free treatment for sexually transmitted diseases and their annual incidence of HIV infection decreased from 18 percent to 3 percent in just over two years (Garcia, 1993). The National Black Women's Health Project (NBWHP), established in 1990, is another example of innovative programming efforts. The CDC is making significant strides in targeted educational programs through the Minority Aids Initiative (MAI), established in 1999. We must continue those efforts which have established creative partnerships with those organizations and institutions that have a natural place in the community. The Down-Low Barbershop Program, initiated in the year 2000 by the Us Helping Us, People Into Living, Inc. organization in Washington, D.C., is an excellent example of this concept. Barbers are trained to be HIV prevention peer educators and workshops are conducted at the barbershops. The intent is to expand this prevention project to beauty salons in order to target women (Krisberg, 2003–2004).

The single most influential resource in the U.S. African American community is the Black Church. It is imperative that the church become more involved in outreach and intervention efforts recognizing that true empowerment comes through teaching of the holy scriptures as given to us in the *New World Translation of the Holy Bible* (1984, p. 1416), Romans 10, verses 14 and 15:

> However, how will they call on him in whom they have not put faith?
> How, in turn, will they put faith in him of whom they have not heard?
> How, in turn, will they hear without someone to preach? How in turn
>   will they preach unless they have been sent forth?

When developing programs, whether secular or faith based, the consumers of the service are an integral part of the design process. Within the African American community, positivism is crucial. Subsequently, the name of the program should be positive and support self-empowerment rather than identify the problem. Program materials should be multicultural and give evidence of an understanding of the different cultural interpretation of common expressions. They should also be Afrocentric by design and reflect our own standards of beauty and color.

An example of this is Rosanna DeMarco and Christine Johnsen's article, "Taking Action in Communities: Women Living with HIV/AIDS Lead the Way," which provides leadership in terms of community-based initiatives that allow women to heal. Through the collaborative efforts of HIV/AIDS organizations, a school of nursing at a university, and women living with HIV/AIDS, a series of educational programs were developed that ultimately empowered women living with HIV/AIDS to end their silence, find meaning in their experience, and develop health strategies that could be implemented in their own communities (DeMarco & Johnsen, 2003). The curriculum developed for two programs, What's in it for Us and Women and HIV: From Silencing to Action, speak directly to the needs of the silent African American woman whose voice must be heard.

REFERENCES

African American Living Legends Series. n.d. Accessed January 2, 2005, from http://www.colapublib.org/bhm/census.html.

American Heritage Dictionary. 3rd ed. 1996. Boston, MA: Houghton Mifflin Company.

Ashante, M. K., and M. Mattison. 1991. *Historical and Cultural Atlas of African Americans.* New York: Macmillan.

Avery, Byllye Y. 1992. "The Health Status of Black Women." In R. Braithwaite and S. E. Taylor (Eds.), *Health Issues in The Black Community* (pp. 35–51). San Francisco, CA: Jossey-Bass.

Billingsley, Andrew. 1992. *Climbing Jacob's Ladder: The Enduring Legacy of African American Families.* New York: Simon & Schuster.

Braithwaite, R. L., and S. E. Taylor (Eds.). 2001. *Health Issues in the Black Community.* 2nd ed. San Francisco, CA: Jossey-Bass.

Browne-Marshall, Gloria J. 2004. "America's Epidemic: HIV/AIDS and People of Color." *Human Rights: Journal of the Section of Individual Rights and Responsibilities,* 31(4): 15. Accessed January 6, 2005, from http:/0-web34.epnet.com.library.daemen.edu/citation.

Centers for Disease Control. March 1995. *Recent Trends in Reported U.S. AIDS Cases.* Rockville, MD.

———. 2003. *HIV/AIDS Surveillance Report 2003,* 15. Atlanta, GA.

———. 2004. *HIV/AIDS Surveillance Report.* Rockville, MD.

Curphey, S. 2003. "Black Women's Mental Health Needs Unmet." *Women's E News.* Accessed January 2, 2005, from http://www.womensenews.org/article.cfm/dyn laid/1392.

Dalton, H. L. 1989. "AIDS in Blackface." *Daedalus,* 118, 205–27.

DeMarco, R, and C. Johnsen. 2003. "Taking Action in Communities: Women Living with HIV/AIDS Lead the Way." *Journal of Community Health Nursing,* 20(1): 51–62.

Freund, P., and McGuire, M. 1991. *Health Issues and the Social Body: Critical Sociology.* Englewood Cliffs, NJ: Prentice Hall.

Garcia, Abigail. Spring 1993. "HIV Positive, Church Negative." *Diatribe.* Berkeley, CA: People of Color News Collective.

Hale, C. B. 1992. "A Demographic Profile of African Americans." In R. Braithwaite and S. E. Taylor (Eds.), *Health Issues in the Black Community* (pp. 6–19). San Francisco, CA: Jossey-Bass.

Health Resources and Services Administration. June 1994. *HIV/AIDS Work Group on Health Care Access Issues for African Americans.* Rockville, MD.

Healthy People 2000 Progress Review for Black Americans. n.d. Accessed January 10, 2005, from Healthy People 2000 Web site http://www.omhrc.gov/omh/healthy 2000book/taboa.htm.

hooks, bell. 1981. *Ain't I a Woman: Black Women and Feminism.* Boston, MA: South End Press.

Jones, D. J, S. Beach, R. Forehand, et al. 2003. "Partner Abuse and HIV Infection: Implications for Psychosocial Adjustment in African American Women." *Journal of Family Violence*, 18(5): 257–68.

Kalichman, S., T. Hunter, and J. Kelly. 1992. "Perceptions of AIDS Suspectability among Minority and Nonminority Women at Risk for HIV Infection." *Journal of Counseling and Clinical Psychology*, 60, 725–32.

Kleinman, A. 1988. *The Illness Narrative: Suffering, Healing and the Human Condition.* New York: Basic Books.

Krisberg, Kim. 2003–2004. "Black Community Groups Confront HIV/AIDS Threat." *Nation's Health*, 33(10): 1.

Land, Helen. 1994. "AIDS and Women of Color." *Families in Society: The Journal of Contemporary Human Services*, 6, 355–61.

Lawson, E. J., and A. Thompson. 1994. "The Health Status of Black Women." In R. Staples (Ed.), *The Black Family: Essays and Studies*. Belmont, CA: Wadsworth.

National Center for Health Statistics. 2003. *National Vital Statistics Report*, 52(9).

New World Translation of the Holy Bible. 1984. Watchtower and Bible Tract Society of New York.

Richie, B. 1994. "AIDS: In Living color." In E. White (Ed.), *Black Women's Health Book: Speaking for Ourselves* (pp. 182–87). Seattle, WA: Seal Press.

Sharp, Saundra. 1993. *Black Women for Beginners*. New York: Writers Readers Publishing.

Smith, L., and S. Thrasher. Spring 1993. "A Practice for Working with Overwhelmed African American Families." *Black Caucus Journal of National Association of Black Social Workers 25th Anniversary Issue*, 1–7.

Staples, Robert. 1994. Social Inequality and Black Sexual Pathology. In R. Staples (Ed.), *The Black Family* (pp. 341–49). Belmont, CA: Wadsworth.

United Nations AIDS (UNAIDS). December 2004. AIDS Epidemic Update.

U.S. Department of Health and Human Services. 1985. *Report of the Secretary's Task Force on Black and Minority Health*. Washington, DC: U.S. Government Printing Office.

World Health Organization. May 2004. *The World Health Report 2004–Changing History*.

Williams, P. B., O. Ekundayo, I. E. Udezulu, and A. Omishakin. 2003. "An Ethnically Sensitive and Gender-Specific HIV/AIDS Assessment of African American Women." *Family Community Health*, 26(2): 108–23.

Williams, Patricia. 1991. "A New Focus on AIDS in Women." *ASM News*, 57(3), 133–34.

Wingood, G. M., and R. J. DiClemente. 1997. "The Effects of an Abusive Partner on Condom Use and Sexual Negotiation Practices of African American Women." *American Journal of Public Health*, 87, 1016–18.

9

African American Women and Depression

FREIDA HOPKINS OUTLAW

When bell hooks (who prefers that her name be spelled with lowercase letters) published *Ain't I a Woman, Black Women and Feminism*, she noted that when beginning the research, she was ridiculed for her concern for the circumstances of Black women in the United States. She reported that one person at a dinner party at which she was discussing the focus of the book laughed and exclaimed, "What is there to say about Black women!" (hooks, 1981). However, more than twenty years later, as the twentieth century closes, there has been increased interest in women's health issues in general, and an organized, focused effort to ensure that women, and especially women of color, are included in all federally sponsored biomedical and behavioral research (Leigh & Jimenez, 2005). The creation of the Office of Women's Health within the U.S. Department of Health and Human Services (DHHS) was an outcome of these endeavors.

Much of the focus on women and women of color's health issues have been stimulated by the changing demographics of the United States, combined with the federal government's requirement that women and minorities be included in all sponsored biomedical and behavioral research. There is emergent support and recognition of the importance of learning about women's health including the influence of race, ethnicity, culture, socioeconomic conditions, and other factors on their health outcomes (Leigh & Jimenez, 2005). Consequently, there have been substantial developments in the study of women and minorities' health and of the correlation of their health to the overall quality of their lives.

However, there continues to be an absence of systematic, reliable empirical national data on the epidemiology of mental disorders among women of color as well as on the prevalence of their use or nonuse of mental health services (Barbee, 1992; Mays et al., 1996, Padget et al., 1998). The invisibility of women of color in mental health research studies has severely limited the empirical data on which to develop evidence-based, race-, ethnicity-, culture-, and gender-specific prevention and intervention clinical and policy strategies. Therefore, this chapter will continue the tradition set by bell hooks (talking about the concerns of Black women) by addressing the issues related to the mental health status of women of African descent using existing literature and empirical data from relevant studies.

In this chapter the term "women of African descent" or "Black women" will be used to refer to those persons whose lineage includes Black ancestors from Africa. This is done to be more inclusive of all women of the African Diaspora. However, unless specifically stated this chapter is primarily focused on African American women, a distinct group of women of African descent who were born and raised in the United States of America. It is the author's belief that their "lived experiences" are different in many aspects, including their history after their forced relocations, from their Caribbean or African sisters who are also women of Black African descent.

HISTORICAL OVERVIEW OF WOMEN OF AFRICAN DESCENT IN THE UNITED STATES

African American women are part of a group whose ancestors were brought to this country unwillingly, beginning in 1619, as slaves to work primarily in the South (Leigh & Jimenez, 2005). Although the number of Africans and African Caribbeans that willingly migrated to this country in the last fifteen years increased significantly, this chapter will as much as possible, focus on African American women born in the United States. (When reporting research findings, it is not always clear who is in the sample.) This level of specificity is important, as recent studies have begun to delineate intragroup variances in many aspects of life within U.S. Black populations and found some of these differences to be more pronounced than intergroup differences between Black and white people.

For example, a recent study found that there were remarkable differences in the prevalence of major mental and physical disorders within Black populations in the United States. African American women were twice as likely as African American men (13.1 percent compared to 7.4 percent) to have experienced a major depression sometime in their lives. Comparatively, only 10 percent of Afro-Caribbean women were found to have experienced a major depression sometime over the course of their lifetime. The resources also noted that African American women had higher rates of both diabetes and high blood pressure than all the other groups of women ("Prevalence of Mental, Physical Disorders," 2004). For instance, Afro-Caribbean people in general have a higher standard of living and better living and social conditions than African Americans, as well as a legacy that is not overshadowed by a long period of enslavement (Gopaul-McNicol, 1993). By comparison, a large percentage of African American women are living in poverty, a condition highly associated with poor mental and physical health. For a number of years the association between African Americans' physical and mental health has been found to be impaired by stress, low socioeconomic status, discrimination, racism, and sexism (Outlaw, 1993; Primm & Gomez, 2005).

Further analysis of health disparities experienced by women, and particularly African American women, supports the inclusion of gender, as well as race, culture, socioeconomic status, and ethnicity, as factors to be understood if we are to develop mental health interventions for this diverse group of women. Presently, the majority of studies of women's mental health have focused on white women's experiences, and therefore are not generalizable to women of other racial and ethnic groups (Woods et al., 1999).

Black women account for over half (18 million) of the nearly 34.7 million (12.3 percent of the total population) black people in this country. Many of these women have claimed African, Caribbean, Native American, and European linkages, with the most common combination (45 percent) of mixtures being African American and white (Leigh & Jimenez, 2005). There is even more heterogeneity further found within this group of African American women due to their regional locations and their cultural and socioeconomic circumstances. For example, a fifth-generation, southern, African American young woman with physician parents will have some similar, but many different, experiences than to an East Coast African American young woman who is a first-generation college student with a single mother. Each will likely have had some experience with discriminatory acts, however, living with educated parents and the influence of regional cultural norms and enriched experiences that are possible when there more monetary resources are available usually create heterogeneity in the experiences and worldview of African American women.

The immigrant population contributes to the diversity found among groups of people of African descent in the United States. Presently, they are estimated to be about 5 percent of the U.S. Black population and are comprised primarily of French-speaking Haitians, non–Spanish speaking Caribbeans, and people from sub-Saharan Africa. According to Leigh and Jimenez (2005), although seldom studied there are marked differences among the Black women in these groups, and these pronounced differences account for variance in their health outcomes.

In the last thirty years there have arisen within America a Black middle class with incomes and educational attainment comparable to that of white middle-class Americans. However there remains a persistent Black underclass (Gates, 2004). Therefore, when considered as a total group, African Americans are disproportionately poor, with 22 percent living below the poverty line. Poverty does not totally determine how a community functions, as it has been noted that poor Black communities often possess "collective efficacy," a factor that can counteract the disabling circumstances associated with poverty (U.S. Department of Health and Human Services, 2001). However, severe poverty is highly associated with long-term hardship, experienced over many generations, which produces many socially negative outcomes, including the widespread and persistent inability to recover. Additionally, poverty in African American communities is highly associated with particular forms of family structure and the emergence of households solely supported by females.

Presently over 54 percent of African American children live in single-parent, predominately female-headed households, with approximately 68 percent of them born to unmarried mothers (Coles & Guy-Sheftall, 2003). This pattern of Black, single, female-headed households has not been the norm historically in the United States. The first detailed data from the 1940 national census found that the predominate structure of Black families with children under 18 years old was the two-parent family (Wilson, 1987). The 1940 census data also documented that Black women who headed households were in most instance widows. In fact, Coles and Guy-Sheftall (2003) noted that as recently as 1960, 78 percent of African Americans with children were married couples.

The structure of the family is significant, as female-headed households currently are highly associated with poor financial assets, impoverished living conditions and other negative sequale associated with poverty. Historically, the core of the African American family structure has been the nuclear family, despite the legacy of slavery. Slaves were noted to work to maintain their family structures as evidenced by their strict marriage taboos, naming practices, and very strict sexual mores that included a restriction on premarital sexual behavior (Davis, 1983). The decline in marriages and high divorce rates are associated with joblessness, rates of incarceration, and premature death experienced disproportionately by Black men. These factors have dramatically changed the structure of many Black families, leading to high rates of poverty among the female heads of households (Coles & Guy-Sheftall, 2003; Wilson, 1987, 1997).

RACE, GENDER, POVERTY, DEPRESSION, AND AFRICAN AMERICAN WOMEN

Poverty is strongly linked with poor health, a risk factor for depression in African American females, who are disproportionately diagnosed with type 2 diabetes, HIV infection, obesity, heart disease, and other chronic medical diseases (deGroot et al., 2003; Gary & Yarandi, 2004; Ginty, 2005). Poor health, while not always an outcome of poverty, is highly correlated with lack of financial and other supportive resources, as well as with environmental factors such as living in substandard housing and continuous exposure to hazards such as chemical toxins and neighborhood violence. These are the lived experiences of many African American women. For example, deGroot et al. (2003) examined the relationship of elements of poverty and depression in African American women at risk for type 2 diabetes. At the beginning of the study, 40 percent of the women were assessed as having a clinical depression and 43 percent were living below the poverty line. They found that unemployment, limited financial resources, lack of home ownership and increased life events were just some of the stressors that predicted depression in this group.

Finally, noting that African American women have double the risk of having a preterm baby as white women, a disparity that has existed for over 50 years, a study was conducted to examine this phenomenon. Orr et al. (2002) measured depressive symptoms in a sample of low-income pregnant African American women receiving prenatal care in a clinic in Baltimore. They found that maternal depressive symptoms in this sample of African American women were independently associated with preterm birth. They also posit that women who develop a major depression during pregnancy are at high risk for experiencing a recurrence of depression over the next five years and longer, and are more likely to develop negative health behaviors such as smoking (Orr et al., 2002). These findings are significant as preterm babies are more likely to develop cognitive, behavioral, social, and mood problems (Le et al., 2004). Therefore, depression in women of childbearing age is profoundly destructive of their physical and mental health as well as of the physical and mental health of their children.

Racism, oppression, and discrimination are stressful events that increase the risk for developing physical and psychiatric illnesses (Billingsley, 1992; Hacker, 1992; Outlaw, 1993). A plethora of studies have shown that African American patients often receive less than optimal technical health care than white American patients, when treated by white physicians (Rask et al., 1994). Cooper-Patrick et al. (1999) also found that African American patients in their study rated their visits to white physicians as "less participatory" than when they saw a physician of their own race. They described the latter as visits in which they were able to participate in the decision making about their care. This finding suggests that patients' perceptions of a positive relationship between themselves and their physician or other health care provider is correlated with positive outcomes, such as patient adherence to treatment.

Racial discrimination has been associated with the health care of Black people as early as the 1800s and has been highly associated with their reluctant use of mental health services (U.S. Department of Health and Human Services, 2001). Several studies have documented that in black communities, in general, there is a healthy distrust of mental health services including psychotherapy and pre-scription of psychotropic medications (Grier & Cobbs, 1968; Comas-Diaz & Greene, 1994; Lawson et al., 1994; Whaley, 2001). Terms such as "cultural paranoia" (Grier & Cobbs, 1968), "healthy cultural paranoia" (Terrell & Ter-rell, 1984), and "cultural mistrust" (Whaley, 2001) are used to describe ways in which African Americans over time learned to protect themselves in what they perceived to be a hostile world. Such protective mechanisms are contextual factors that are uniquely related to the experiences of African Americans and are related to their experiences of racial discrimination, economic exploitation, and oppression (Boyd-Franklin, 1989; Jackson & Mustillo, 2001).

Mistrust and suspicion among African Americans of the health care system and the mental health system in particular, are rooted in the history of mis-treatment and misdiagnosis of African Americans that, to some extent, still exist in psychiatric treatment today. For example, a recent study of prescribing pat-terns of outpatient psychiatrists, while improved since the 1990s, found that African Americans with psychotic disorders are less likely to be prescribed atypical antipsycotic medications than either Hispanic or white people (Daumit et al., 2003). Atypical antipsyotics are currently considered the first line treat-ment for psychotic disorders, interfere less with cognitive function, and cause fewer negative side-effects than typical antipsycotics. However, they are more costly than typical antipsychotic medications.

Additionally, treatment for mental health disorders among members of African American communities is associated with police, involuntary hospitalization (Meinert et al., 2003), and the use of more restrictive forms of interventions, such as seclusion and mechanical restraint (Outlaw & Lowery, 1994), chemical restraint, and treatment environments devoid of African American therapists. The lack of therapists of African descent suggests that the cultural sensitivity needed for the appropriate assessment, diagnosis, and treatment of African American women with depression may be severely compromised (Barbee, 1992).

In general, mental health programs have traditionally ignored race, ethnicity, culture, and gender when treating African American women. Barbee (1992) noted that the research-derived evidence that guides and informs mental health practice is a contextual and is not generally descriptive of the experiences of African American women with depression. Thus, the treatment of depression in African American women, despite the association with poor physical health outcomes, diminished quality of life and negative impact on parenting, is woefully inadequate and uninformed by evidence-based research and scholarly clinical practice.

CONSTRUCTING A PICTURE OF DEPRESSION IN AFRICAN AMERICAN WOMEN: CULTURAL, SOCIAL, AND OTHER RELEVANT FACTORS

A major mental health problem throughout the world, depression has been projected by the World Health Organization to become, by 2020, the most devastating illness in the world (Choenarom et al., 2005). Depression, from a clinical point of view, has been described in the DSM IV-TR (American Psychiatric Association [APA], 2000) as an interrelated set of symptoms, with the most common being feelings of loss of interest and pleasure in activities, and a depressed or sad mood. Other core symptoms of depression include helplessness, hopelessness, difficulty concentrating on a task, frequent thoughts of death, feelings of guilt and worthlessness, weight loss or gain, agitation and irritability, decreased desire for sex, pain, withdrawal and isolation, problems at work, and physical symptoms (APA, 2000). There are also levels of depression ranging from mild to severe. Depression is an illness that involves the mind, body, and spirit and is different from a passing "blue mood." It is not a sign, however, of personal weakness or a condition that can be willed or wished away. Although the exact mechanisms are not clearly known, there is evidence that neurotransmitter bioamines play a role in the transmission and regulation of neurological pathways, and selected hormones, play a part in depression. However there are strong indications that there are social and cultural factors involved in an individual becoming depressed (Kleinman & Good, 1985).

Cultural and social factors have an influence on mental illness but vary by disorder. However they have been found to be heavily associated with the causation and prevalence of major depression (U.S. Department of Health and Human Services, 2001). While psychiatric disorders such as bipolar disorder, panic disorder, and schizophrenia show global consistency in symptoms and prevalence and have been found to have high heritablity, studies have found much less heritablity for major depression (DHHS, 2001). Current evidence from National Institute of Mental Health (NIMH) studies strongly suggests that social, economic, and cultural factors such as poverty, exposure to violence, and other stressful factors such as racial and gender discrimination have a very direct casual role in episodes of major depression (DHHS, 2001).

There is heterogeneity among African American women, however as a group they are disproportionately poor, making them at risk for experiencing a major depression (Gary & Yarandi, 2004). Although middle-class African American women can have a major depression, as they are exposed to social factors such as racial discrimination and oppression related to gender, several studies have found that income, age, marital status, and education level are associated with depression in Black women (Scarinci et al., 2002). That is, Scarinci et al. (2002) found that the higher the yearly household income and education level of the Black women in their study, the lower the depression rate. They also noted higher levels of depression in younger Black women and women who were not married, compared to those who were married or living with an intimate partner. In a similar finding, Woods et al. (1999) found in their study that depression among Black women was the result of a number of negative life events, con- flicted network size, and low levels of religious activity. However, education mitigated developing depression in this group. Warren (1997) found that African American women who were highly stressed experienced high levels of de- pression, while those who had high levels of social support experienced lower levels of depression. Taken together, these studies have identified as buffers against depression among Black women low levels of stress and social support.

Acknowledging that poverty, unemployment, living alone, and other negative social conditions are highly associated with depression in African American women, what are some of the internal and external cultural norms that are extreme mundane stressors that make Black women as a group more vulnerable to depression?

Pierce (1975) defines extreme mundane stressors as those daily encounters that are persistent and caustic that are constantly wearing on the person's mind, body, and spirit. He suggests that Black people in this country experience mundane stress as a daily lived experience. There are, for example, external to the group mainstream norms for women that define them as fragile, permissive, vulnerable, and submissive, yet Black women as a group historically have had to be strong, resilient, and self-affirming in order to sustain themselves and their families (Comas-Diaz & Greene, 1994). For as has been documented, no other racial, ethnic, cultural, or religious group of women in this country has experienced the degree of stereotyping, degradation, hardship, and discrimination as Black women (Ladner, 1971; McGoldrick et al., 1991). Black women are phenotypi- cally, emotionally, and culturally diverse from white women, yet they are often marginalized when they do not conform to mainstream group norms, that is, norms associated with white women (Greene, 1994).

The marginalization originated during slavery when, to justify the subjugation of Black women to the harsh conditions of forced labor, they were not included in the accepted definitions of womanhood (Coles & Guy-Sheftall, 2003). In order to survive such a hostile environment with demeaning images and stereotypes, a widely held coping strategy subscribed to by Black women was the notion of the cultural imperative to "be strong" through it all.

The idea of being strong as a characteristic of Black women is accepted as a cultural imperative among Black people in general, and as a widely held belief among white women. Feminist filmmaker Aisha Shahidah Simmons, while talking about her documentary *NO!*, an exploration of the silence in Black communities about the intraracial rape of Black women, said that very often white women will express surprise during discussions about the film that Black women can be raped (personnel conversation, April 2005). She stated white women consistently say that they "thought Black women were too strong to be raped."

The idea of being strong has been reported by Black West Indian women living in Canada. They identified "being strong" as a basic social process that helps them to manage depression as a minority group in a Eurocentric society (Schreiber et al., 2000). For these women, being strong was a cultural imperative that has been accepted and espoused from one generation to the next, and has been a specific cultural norm of Black women, distinct from norms for white women. In the study conducted by Schreiber et al. (2000), one Black woman stated "I think Black women are stronger than whites. They've been, I mean, I'm talking about going back with generations so you were raised to be, you know, the strength of the home, the mother" (p. 39). It would appear that the idea of being strong is highly associated with motherhood, and, metaphorically, with being the nurturer and protector of the race, very awesome tasks.

In order to protect the race, often being strong for many Black women means that they are keeping personal issues inside the family while maintaining a "stiff upper lip" (Meinert et al., 2003) about any emotional problems they are experiencing (p. 24). Coles and Guy-Sheftall (2003) discuss this phenomenon of not wanting to "air their dirty linen in public." As a result, Black women are often silent about physical and sexual abuse perpetuated on them by Black males, as a way of being strong. This collective cultrual norm held by many Black women allows Black communities to avoid focusing on the intersection of gender and race, allowing the race problem to be male centered (Coles & Guy-Sheftall, 2003).

Black women experience a type of "double bind" where keeping silent about egregious abuse by Black men places them at high risk for depression, but exposing Black men who physically and sexually abuse them may seem to them disloyal to their communities, again placing them at risk for depression. The double bind theory posits when as individual experiences two conflicting messages from the same person (the second through body language) from which they must make a choice that will result in a sanction or punishment, negative emotional consequences for the individual are the usual outcome (Foley, 1974).

Others have described the phenomenon of "being strong" and the subsequent sequel, "being silent" about emotional problems, as distinct cultural phenomena found among Black women. Mays et al. (1996), in their discussion of the service utilization patterns of African American women, stated that solving intrapsychic problems is thought by many Black women to be part of what it means to be independent and self-reliant, components of being strong.

Meinert et al. (2003) identified similar attitudes among the African American women that they studied who espoused self-help and the belief that as African American women they must "keep on keeping on," a strong cultural value. This emphasis on keeping on and not taking care of self has been documented in the literature as being a form of behavior exhibited by Black women that is connected to their well-documented delay, and sometimes avoidance of, seeking treatment for both physical and mental health illnesses. Again, the "keeping on" behaviors are highly associated with being strong in order that they might take care of their families.

TREATMENT OF AFRICAN AMERICAN WOMEN WITH DEPRESSION: RELIGION, THE BLACK CHURCH AND CULTURALLY COMPETENT PROVIDERS

Religion, the Black Church and Depression in Black Women

During a psychoeducation program sponsored by the United Methodist Christian Women's Society, Outlaw and Bradley (2003), surveyed the group of participants concerning their knowledge about and experiences with depression. There were forty-one African American women in a group of sixty-two women. The African American women ranged in age from 27 to 79 with a mean age of 51. They used a variety of words to describe depression including "down, feeling low," "feeling bad," "unhappy," "blue," "not caring," "crying," "when I stop singing," and "not facing reality." These descriptors of depression were congruent with what Barbee (1992) in her study found to be a distinctive language and wording for depression used by the African American women. She suggested that the nomenclature used by the women is culturally constructed with the genesis of understanding depression rooted in their experiences with blues music (Barbee, 1992), a musical genre that talks about misery and pain, a symbolic expression of feelings associated with depression. It is at the conceptual level of cultural experience that therapists can connect authentically with the pain of their client, especially if there are racial, ethnic, and cultural discordance. When therapists are learning to work with clients of various racial, ethnic, and cultural groups, they must elicit the worldview of the clients instead of discounting it, in order to form an authentic therapeutic relationship across racial, ethnic, cultural, and socioeconomic lines (Barbee, 1992; Boyd-Franklin, 1989; Outlaw, 1993; Warren, 1997).

Seventeen of the forty-one women in the Outlaw and Bradley (2003) survey had received some form of treatment, including medication, therapy, hospitalization, or a combination, for their depression. Another five women said that they refused treatment because "they did not know any better." When asked "who they would prefer to get help from," the majority said that they would like to have a combination of a psychoeducation and traditional therapy group comprised of women such as themselves. Rapmund (1999) suggested that depression in women is a subjective, context-related experience, therefore women need to talk about the context in which it takes place. He advocates treatment that allows women to tell their stories, which gives them the voice to describe how they perceive their experiences. The African American women in the Outlaw and Bradley survey, like the women in the Rapmund study, were asking for more information sessions about depression. The African American women in the Outlaw and Bradley (2003) survey also requested a venue to share their personal stories as Black women with each other, a way of having a collective voice about their unique experiences of depression.

Interestingly, 70 percent of the African American women in the Outlaw and Bradley (2003) survey said they would not like to get help for their depression from a member of the clergy, and 57.6 percent said they would not like to get help from a family member. This finding is divergent from what is often found in the literature about whom Black women turn to for mental health support. Divergent findings such as this one add to the empirical data needed to support the development of evidence-based interventions. Empirical data may challenge traditional ways of thinking about what constitutes a church-based intervention; however, these data can be used to develop church-based interventions that support the unique mental health needs of African American women who as a group have been the foundation of the organized Black Church. It has been stated that "if it wasn't for women, you [African Americans] wouldn't have a church!" (Coles & Guy-Sheftall, 2003, p. 110).

The Black Church is the most powerful and important institution in the Black community. However, some of the institutional practices and ideological tenets have not empowered women, and thus have been thought by some to be counter-productive to the positive psychological development of women. The Black Church, having been modeled on white Protestant religious traditions, has a history of male dominance, best symbolized by the practice of forbidding the ordination of women to preach from the pulpit. Presently, there are a group of clergy whose theological values, beliefs, and teachings are compelling them to focus on gender equality, liberation theology, and the particular experiences of African American women (Coles & Guy-Sheftall, 2003), including their mental health concerns such as depression. With this progressive movement in the Black Church, perhaps the silence about mental health issues will be eradicated, making the church a vital partner in serving the mental health needs of the Black community.

A great opportunity exists to have the Black Church as an institution become better imbedded in the collective psyche of Black people, which is often de-scribed by them as "a place of refuge in a mighty storm" (Coles & Guy-Sheftall, 2003), take leadership in this endeavor. It would allow the Black Church to lead the movement in developing evidence for needed culturally specific mental health interventions that are therapeutic for Black people. To date, there is a dearth of evidence-based practices for the treatment of mental illness in Black populations in general (Betancourt et al., 2005; Hyde et al., 2003), and among Black women in particular (Barbee, 1994; DHHS, 2001).

Investigators such as Taylor and Chatters (1988) and Caldwell et al. (1995) found that African American women's religious participation, church atten-dance, church membership, and subjective religiosity were significantly related to their receipt of support for emotional concerns from church members. While these are important findings, the transition from science to service needs to be tracked. One promising community-based church sponsored conference raising awareness about suicide and the greatest risk factor, depression, is the annual conference on Suicide and the Black Church: The Silent Storm, sponsored by the Healing Center in Memphis, Tennessee, a church led by the pastor Dr. William Young. This conference began as a result of a very painful moment in the church's history. In March 2002, a female member of the church went on the grounds, positioned herself under the cross, and committed suicide. The conference is a bold step and part of a new movement among innovative Black churches to confront problems that are rampant but generally ignored in Black communities because of stigma about mental illness, substance abuse, suicide, and HIV/AIDS.

Cultural Competence and Presentation of Depressive Symptoms by Black Women

Health care professionals have to explore and be more culturally aware of and competent in identifying and understanding the root of the symptoms of the patients that they are serving. The genesis of some of the underreporting of depression in African Americans is the difference in the presentation of symptoms in this group (Gallo et al., 1998). African American women may not present with a pronounced depressed mood; rather, they may have more exaggerated symptoms such as fatigue, "sick and tired of being sick and tired" (a very popular phrase used by African American women), and loss of concentration (Brown et al., 2003; Gary & Yarandi, 2004). There have also been noted discrepancies in the presentations of white women and Black women around the symptom of weight gain. In general, when depressed, white women lose weight because they have decreased appetites, while Black women tend to gain weight.

TRENDS IN SOCIAL AND PUBLIC POLICY INFLUENCING THE TREATMENT OF AFRICAN AMERICAN WOMEN WITH DEPRESSION

The creation of the Office of Minority Health in 1987 and the creation of the National Institutes of Health (NIH) Revitalization Act of 1993 both mandated that women and minorities be included in all NIH-sponsored research, including phase III clinical trials (Leigh & Jimenez, 2005). These two initiatives have influenced the movement to develop specific scientific knowledge to inform prevention, assessment, and intervention and treatment strategies for African American women with mental disorders, such as depression. Concurrently, the federal government is emphasizing the development of strategies by which to effectively translate research findings into practice, since it has been known for some time that research findings are seldom implemented in practice settings without significant modifications.

The National Institute of Mental Health (NIMH) currently is focusing on translating science into service through the implementation of evidence-based practices at the state level. To this end, policy issues being implemented at state levels are focused on best practices, evidence-based practices and cultural competence. These policy decisions drive how resources are spent. For example, the Tennessee Department of Mental Health and Developmental Disabilities (TDMHDD) has disseminated Best Practice Guidelines for Children and Adolescents and Adults to providers including the twenty-two Community Mental Health Agencies and the five Regional Mental Health Institutes that are run by the state. This was one step in a series of strategies to move best evidence into the clinical arena.

These policy initiatives at both the national and state level will determine regional and local approaches to implementing culturally specific strategies. For example, the TDMHDD Best Practice Guidelines noted that cultural and ethnic differences in presentations of symptoms could cause underdiagnosis or misdiagnosis of depression. There are other references to the influence of gender, race and ethnicity, and the treatment of depression, anxiety, and bipolar disorder in adults. However, in future guidelines more attention will need to be paid to gender and culturally specific treatment for depression that is gender, racially, culturally, and ethnically specific.

As Mechanic (1999) noted, we cannot assume that mental health treatments that are not effective are benign. An extreme example of a mental health intervention that was not benign is the lobotomy. Less dramatic, but just as critical, is any treatment that does not produce positive outcomes and contributes to prolonged client suffering. It is known that mental health treatments that are not gender, racially, culturally, and ethnically specific have not demonstrated efficacy, and thus have prolonged suffering experienced by clients. For African American women with depression, this prolonged suffering has implications for their emotional and physical health. The creation of the Office of Minority Health; the National Institutes of Health Revitalization Act; and efforts of state governments to implement polices supporting treatment of depression and other mental disorders that are culturally appropriate, by providers that are culturally competent and using racially, ethnically, culturally, and gender specific interventions, are examples of intelligent public policy.

SUMMARY

The treatment of depression in African American women is not where it once was nor where it needs to be, but the development of evidence-based practices that are racially, ethnically, culturally, and gender specific holds great promise for the high number of African American women who suffer from depression. Additionally, the mobilization of resources in the Black community, such as progressive Black churches, is a venue that holds promise for intervening effectively in the overrepresentation of depression in African American women.

Depression can be treated successfully. According to Dr. Lewis-Hall, more than 80 percent of people with clinical depression can recover and resume normal, productive lives (Healthy Place, 2005). However, as suggested by Le et al. (2003), the policy initiative that needs to be implemented is the promotion of a national agenda to prevent major depression in all women.

REFERENCES

American Psychiatric Association. 2000. *Diagnostic and Statistical Manual of Mental Disorders, Fourth Edition, Text Revision.* Washington, DC: Author.

Barbee, E. 1992. "African American Women and Depression. A Review and Critique of the Literature." *Archives of Psychiatric Nursing,* 6, 257–265.

———. 1994. "Healing Time: The Blues in African-American Women." *Health Care for Women International,* 15, 53–60.

Betancourt, J. R., A. R. Green, J. E. Carrillo, and E. R. Park. 2005. "Cultural Competence and Health Care Disparities: Key Perspectives and Trends." *Health Affairs,* 24, 499–505.

Billingsley, A. 1992. *Climbing Jacob's Ladder: The Enduring Legacy of African American Families.* New York: Simon & Schuster.

Boyd-Franklin, N. 1989. *Black Families in Therapy: A Multi-systems Approach.* New York: Guilford Press.

Brown, C., C. Abe-Kim, and C. Barrio. 2003. "Depression in Ethnically Diverse Women: Implications for Treatment in Primary Care Settings." *Professional Psychology: Research and Practice,* 34, 10–19.

Caldwell, C. H., L. M. Chatters, A. Billingsley, and R. J. Taylor. 1995. "Church-based Support Programs for Elderly Black Adults: Congregational and Clergy Characteristics." In M. A. Kimble, S. H. McFadden, J. W. Ellor, and J. J. Seeber (Eds.), *Aging, Spirituality, and Religion: A Handbook* (pp. 306–324). Minneapolis, MN: Augsburg Fortress.

Choenarom, C., R. Williams, and B. M. Hagerty. 2005. "The Role of Sense of Belonging and Social Support on Stress and Depression in Individuals with Depression." *Archives of Psychiatric Nursing,* 19, 18–29.

Coles, J. B., and B. Guy-Sheftall. 2003. *Gender Talk: The Struggle for Women's Equality in African American Communities.* New York: Random House.

Comas-Diaz, L., and B. Greene. 1994. *Women of Color: Integrating Ethnic and Gender Identities in Psychotherapy.* New York: Guilford Press.

Cooper-Patrick, L., J. Gallo, J. Gonzales, H. Vu, N. Powe, C. Nelson, and D. Ford. 1999. "Race, Gender, and Partnership in the Patient-physician Relationship." *Journal of the American Medical Association,* 282, 583–589.

Daumit, G. L., R. M. Crum, E. Guallar, N. R. Powe, A. B. Primm, D. M. Steinwachs, and D. E. Ford. 2003. "Outpatient Prescriptions for Atypical Antipsychotics for African Americans, Hispanics, and Whites in the United States." *Archives of General Psychiatry,* 60, 121–128.

Davis, A. Y. 1983. *Women, Race and Class.* New York: Vintage Books.

deGroot, M., W. Auslander, J. Williams, M. Sherraden, and D. Haire-Joshu. 2003. "Depression and Poverty among African American Women at Risk for Type 2 Diabetes." *Annals of Behavioral Medicine,* 25, 172–181.

Foley, V. 1974. *An Introduction to Family Therapy.* New York: Greene & Stratton.

Gallo, J., L. Cooper-Patrick, and S. Lesikar. 1998. "Depressive Symptoms of Whites and African Americans Aged 60 Years and Older." *Journal of Gerontology: Psychological Sciences,* 53B, 277–286.

Gallo, J. J., S. Marino, D. Ford, and J. C. Anthony. 1995. "Filters on the Pathway to Mental Health Care, II. Sociodemographic Factors." *Psychological Medicine,* 25, 1149–1160.

Gary, F., and H. Yarandi. 2004. "Depression among Southern Rural African American Women: A Factor Analysis of the Beck Depression Inventory—11." *Nursing Research,* 53, 251–259.

Gates, H. L. 2004. *America Behind the Color Line: Dialogues with African Americans*. New York: Warner Books.

Ginty, M. M. 2005. "Black Women at Higher Risk for Major Diseases." *Women's E-News*. Available online at http://www.womensenews.org/article.cfm/dyn/aid/2197 /context/archive.

Gopaul-McNicol, S. 1993. *Working with West Indian Families*. New York: Guilford Press.

Greene, B. 1994. "African American Women." In L. Comas-Diaz and B. Greene (Eds.), *Women of Color: Integrating Ethnic and Gender Identities in Psychotherapy* (pp. 30–71). New York: Guilford Press.

Grier, W. H., and P. M. Cobbs. 1968. *Black Rage*. New York: Basic Books.

Hacker, A. 1992. *Two Nations: Black and White, Separate, Hostile, and Unequal*. New York: Ballantine Press.

The Healing Center. June 2005. *Second Suicide and the Black Church Conference II: The Silent Storm*. Memphis, TN. Dr. William Young, Pastor.

Healthy Place. 2005. "Fighting 'the Blues' in African Americans." Available online at http.//www.healtyhplace.com/communities/depression/minorities9.asp.

hooks, b. 1981. *Ain't I a Woman: Black Women and Feminism*. Boston: South End Press.

Hyde, P., K. Falls, J. A. Morris, and S. K. Schoenwald. 2003. *Turning Knowledge into Practice: A Manual for Behavioral Health Administrators and Practitioners about Understanding and Implementing Evidence-based Practices*. Boston, MA: The Technical Assistance Collaborative, Inc.

Jackson, P. B., and S. Mustillo. 2001. "I Am Woman: The Impact of Social Identities on African American Women's Mental Health." *Women and Health*, 32, 33–59.

Kleinman, A., and B. Good. 1985. "Introduction: Culture and Depression." In A. Kleinman and B. Good (Eds.), *Culture and Depression* (pp. 1–33). Berkley, CA: University of California Press.

Ladner, J. A. 1971. *Tomorrow's Tomorrow: The Black Woman*. Garden City, NY: Anchor Books.

Lawson, W. B., N. Hepler, J. Halladay, and B. Cuffel. 1994. "Race As a Factor, Inpatient and Outpatient Admissions and Diagnosis." *Hospital and Community Psychiatry*, 45, 72–74.

Le, N., R. Muñoz, C. Ippen, and J. Stoddard. 2003. "Treatment Is Not Enough: We Must Prevent Major Depression in Women." *Prevention and Treatment*, 6, art. 10.

Leigh, W. A., and M. A. Jimenez. 2005. *Women of Color Health Data Book* (2nd Ed.). Bethesda, MD: National Institutes of Health, Office of Research on Women's Health. Accessed online June 2005 at http://www4.od.nih/gov/orwh/wocEnglish 202.pdf.

Mays, V. M., C. H. Caldwell, and J. S. Jackson. 1996. "Mental Health Symptoms and Service Utilization Patterns of Help-seeking among African American Women." In H. W. Neighbors and J. S. Jackson (Eds.), *Mental Health in Black America* (pp. 161–176). Thousand Oaks, CA: Sage Publications.

McGoldrick, M., C. Anderson, and F. Walsh (Eds.). 1991. "Women in Families: A Framework for Family Therapy." In M. McGoldrick, N. Garcia-Preto, P. Hines, and E. Lee (Eds.), *Ethnicity and Women* (pp. 169–199). New York: W. W. Norton Co.

Mechanic, D. 1999. *Mental Health and Social Policy: The Emergence of Managed Care* (4th Ed.). Boston: Allyn and Bacon.

Meinert, J., M. Blehar, K. Peindl, A. Neal-Barnett, and K. Wisner. 2003. "Recruitment of African American Women into Mental Health Research Studies." *Academic Psychiatry*, 27, 21–28.

Orr, S. T., A. J. Sherman, and C. B. Prince. 2002. "Maternal Prenatal Depression Symptoms and Spontaneous Pre-term Births among African-American Women in Baltimore, Maryland." *American Journal of Epidemiology,* 156, 797–802.

Outlaw, F. H. 1993. "Stress and Coping: The Influence of Racism on the Cognitive Appraisal Processing of African Americans." *Issues in Mental Health Nursing,* 14, 399–409.

Outlaw, F., and P. Bradley. February 21, 2003. "Coping with Women's Stressors—Depression." Presented at Bethel African Americans Women's Health Symposium, San Antonio, TX.

Outlaw, F. H., and B. J. Lowery. 1994. "An Attributional Study of Seclusion and Restraint of Psychiatric Patients." *Archives of Psychiatric Nursing,* 8, 69–77.

Padget, D. K., C. P. Harman, B. J. Burns, and H. J. Schlesinger. 1998. "Women and Outpatient Mental Health Services." In B. L. Levin, A. K. Blanch, and A. Jennings (Eds.), *Women's Mental Health Services: A Public Health Perspective* (pp. 34–54). Thousand Oaks, CA: Sage.

Pierce, C. 1975. "The Mundane Extreme Environment and Its Effect on Learning." In S. G. Brainard (Ed.), *Learning Disabilities: Issues and Recommendations for Research* (pp. 1–23). Washington, DC: Institute of Education.

"Prevalence of Mental, Physical Disorders Varies Within U.S. Black Populations." 2004. *Women's Health Weekly.* News RX.com and News RX.net. Accessed online February 12, 2004, from http://www.lexis.com/research/dellprevalence_of_mental_physical .pdf.

Primm, A., and M. Gomez. 2005. "The Impact of Mental Health on Chronic Disease." In L. A. Daniels (Ed.), *The State of Black America: Prescriptions for Change* (pp. 63–73). New York: National Urban League.

Rapmund, V. J. 1999. "A Story Around the Role of Relationships in the World of a 'Depressed' Woman and the Healing Process." *Contemporary Family Therapy,* 21(2): 239–266.

Rask, K., M. Williams, R. Parker, and S. McNagny. 1994. "Obstacles Predicting Lack of a Regular Provider and Delays in Seeking Care for Patients at an Urban Public Hospital." *Journal of the American Medical Association,* 271, 1931–1933.

Scarinci, I. C., B. M. Beech, W. Nauman, K. W. Kovach, L. Pugh, and B. Fapohunda. 2002. "Depression, Socioeconomic Status, Age, and Marital Status in Black Women: A National Study." *Ethnicity and Disease,* 12, 421–428.

Schreiber, R., P. Stern, and C. Wilson. 2000. "Being Strong: How Black West-Indian, Canadian Women Manage Depression and its Stigma." *Image: Journal of Nursing Scholarship,* 32, 39–45.

Taylor, R., and L. Chatters. 1988. "Church Members as a Source of Informal Social Support." *Review of Religious Research,* 30, 193–203.

Terrell, F., and S. Terrell. 1984. "Race of Counselor, Client Sex, Cultural Mistrust Level, and Premature Termination from Counseling among Black Clients." *Journal of Counseling Psychology,* 31, 371–375.

U.S. Department of Health and Human Services. 2001. *Mental Health: Culture, Race and Ethnicity—A Supplement to Mental Health: A Report of the Surgeon General.* Rockville, MD: U.S. Department of Health and Human Services, Office of Surgeon General.

Warren, B. J. 1997. "Depression, Stressful Life Events, Social Support and Self-esteem in Middle Class African American Women." *Archives of Psychiatric Nursing,* 11, 107–117.

Whaley, A. 2001. "Cultural Mistrust and Mental Health Services for African Americans: A Review and Meta-analysis." *The Counseling Psychologist,* 29, 513–531.

Wilson, W. J. 1987. *The Truly Disadvantaged: The Inner City, and the Underclass, and Public Policy."* Chicago: University of Chicago Press.

———. 1997. *When Work Disappears: The World of the Urban Poor.* New York: Vintage Books.

Woods, N. F., E. M. Lentz, E. Mitchell, and L. D. Oakley. 1999. "Depressed Mood and Self-esteem in Young Asians, Black, and White Women in America." In C. Fordes, A. E. Hunter, and B. Burns (Eds.), *Readings in the Psychology of Women: Dimensions of the Female Experience* (pp. 328–339). Boston: Allyn and Bacon.

10

Homeless Women: Caught in a Web of Poverty

JUANITA K. HUNTER

The complexity of the modern-day homeless problem has deepened over the past ten years. According to the Stewart B. McKinney Homeless Assistance Act of 1987, a homeless person is one who lacks a fixed, regular, and adequate residence. Public or privately operated shelters or other temporary residences are not considered fixed and regular within this definition (Hombs, 2001, p. 51; P.L. 100-77, 1987). Homelessness has been typically associated with individuals who have utilized all available resources for income and housing, or those without a tangible support system. Few individuals elect this nomad way of life. Historically, single men previously comprised the bulk of the "identified" homeless.

Literature continues to document an unprecedented increase in the numbers of homeless individuals and particularly, single mothers with children. Nationwide, the majority of this group are African American single women. The overhaul of the public welfare system in the 1990s left many individuals previously eligible for monetary benefits with no means of support. These homeless women and children experience frequent episodes of shelter living during a given year. The plight of these individuals should be of concern to the broader African American community. Structural problems within the society such as, housing shortages, deinstitutionalization policies, changes in the industrial economy, failed educational systems, racism, and inadequate income supports create the conditions that place people at risk. "The problem is fundamental. The persisting spectacle of homeless people on American streets is a continuing indictment of our collective failure to make the basic ingredients of civilized society accessible to all citizens" (Breakey, 1997, p. 156).

There is a paucity of information that specifically addresses homelessness among African American women. In spite of major economic and social gains,

African Americans still continue to face persistent, discriminatory, and access barriers to the many resources that would enable their complete self-sufficiency and self-actualization. The African American homeless woman confronts these same realities and biases without benefit of a stable home environment and buttress against these challenges.

BACKGROUND

Homelessness is not a new phenomenon for African Americans and can be traced throughout their history. The Africans were brought to America in chains, were countryless and homeless, and were not recognized as persons in their own right. Black enslaved in the United States were bought and sold as commodities. Those enslaved were found both in the north and south, however, the largest concentration was in the South. They could not own property and their place of residence was entirely dependent upon the slave master who owned them. Any attempt to escape often lead to sale to another slave owner, torture, or possibly death.

The end of the Civil War and the Emancipation Proclamation removed some of the restrictions on the mobility of those formerly enslaved. However, the attitudes, laws, and discriminatory practices enacted and enforced in both North and South during Reconstruction, were the driving forces for former slaves to move both north and west to seek true "freedom," and new ways of working and living. The post–Civil War migration brought a steady stream of African Americans to northern cities, and this trend increased during World War II. During this period, some became homeless through loss of family ties, when husbands or other family members preceded them to the northern cities. This significant migration of Blacks increased transiency and homelessness. The Underground Railroad and its supporters provided much of the assistance needed for those in transit. African American women such as Sojourner Truth were strong leaders who spearheaded this movement.

During that era, there was no significant social welfare "safety net" to protect individuals and families from catastrophe. In conjunction with these phenomena, major changes were necessitated in the daily lives of those in transit, as the traditional ways of earning a living, habitation, and social interaction drastically changed in an urban versus their familiar rural community. Urban housing patterns did not enhance the close-knit relationships to which many were accustomed to, in a plantation lifestyle, and thus the familiar extended family and kinship support systems were eroded or severed. However, the experiences of slavery had fostered a strong kinship among those enslaved, and the religious basis of their subculture softened this new existence. The great migration started in 1915 and the proportion of Blacks living in the North and West increased to 23.8 percent by 1940 (Myrdal, 1944). By the late nineteenth century, homelessness was institutionalized within the skid rows of American cities.

The number of homeless persons increased until the late 1920s, when technological changes drastically reduced the demand for unskilled labor (Rossi, 1989). Soup kitchens and bread lines were a community response and attempted to address the problem. With the advent of the Great Depression in the 1930s, homelessness greatly increased. As had previously occurred during World War I, World War II reduced the homeless population. The permanent unemployed of the 1930s virtually disappeared during this period. After World War II, the skid rows were identified as a collection of cheap hotels, restaurants, bars, employment agencies, and churches. African Americans were generally not included in this grouping, nor were they visible, except in certain religious missions.

After World War II, homelessness increased as a result of major changes in housing patterns that included, the movement of middle class Caucasian families to the suburbs, demise of federal support for low-income housing programs, and a dramatic decrease in affordable housing in urban areas. In addition, the end of the War on Poverty and similar programs for addressing social and economic inequities decreased community support for indigent individuals (Hunter, 1995).

SCOPE OF THE PROBLEM

Homelessness has clearly taken on new dimensions in the twenty-first century. The distressing prediction that the problem will continue to increase in severity and scope seems destined to become a reality (Hatton, 2001; Bassuk et al. 1996; U.S. Conference of Mayors, 1997). Further, the majority of homeless persons in large urban areas are now African American with increasing numbers of women (Burt & Cohen, 1989; Breakey et al., 1989). The systemic, structural, and economic forces that create a disproportionate number of poor female-headed households must be considered in any discussion of contemporary homelessness (Bassuk, 1993). Some scholars have demonstrated a link between business and governmental decisions and the increase of homelessness in the United States (Lyon-Callo, 2000). Hopper et al. (1985) cite the increasing globalization of capital, deindustrialization, while other authors have included the growth of temporary labor, declining union membership, institutional racism, and gentrification in the name of community development as major influences (Marcuse, 1989; Williams, 1996). While an accurate number of homeless persons has yet to be quantified, current estimates of the homeless range from 250,000 to some 3 to 4 million. Homeless families now comprise approximately 35 to 50 percent of the homeless group and 67 percent in New York City (U.S. Conference of Mayors, 2003; Luck et al., 2002; Percy, 1995; Hatton, 2001; Redlener, 1999).

The growth of female-headed households living in poverty increases the potential for homelessness (Bassuk, 1993). One in five children in the United States live in poverty, and the fastest growing subgroup within the homeless population are single women with children (National Coalition for the Homeless [NCH], 2001; Bassuk et al., 1997; U.S. Conference of Mayors, 2003; Wright et al., 1998, Chapter 5; Interagency Council on the Homeless, 1991; Burg, 1994). Eighty-five percent of homeless children are headed by single mothers, and 41 percent of these children are aged one to five (Redlener, 1999; Better Homes Fund, 1999). More than half of homeless children are under six years of age. In spite of these trends, the populations studied have been predominantly male (Skelly et al., 1990). Consequently, we know very little about homeless women and, particularly, African American homeless women (Goering et al., 1990).

CAUSES OF HOMELESSNESS

Contemporary homelessness is a multifaceted problem that results from several interconnecting factors, primarily, a lack of affordable housing and poverty (NCH, 2001). Economic conditions, during periods of war, natural disasters, and catastrophies increase the number of homeless. In a survey of twenty-five major cities in 2003, the U.S. Conference of Mayors found that unemployment and lack of affordable housing lead the list of causes of homelessness (U.S. Conference of Mayors, 2003). In today's rapidly changing society, technology, loss of unskilled jobs, lack of education, and poor preparation for the job market are viewed as major contributors to homelessness. Contemporary homelessness is at an all time high (Prentice, 1993), and the consequences disproportionately affect African American women.

Risk factors of an increased divorce rate, substance use, single parenting, personal crises, and domestic violence predispose many more women to homelessness. These risk factors are particularly significant for minority women who live in poverty and are at high risk for victimization by violence (Browne, 1993). Social problems such as the epidemic of teenage pregnancy, more single-parent families, and substance abuse may increase the numbers of homeless (Breakey et al., 1989; Bassuk, 1993; Wagner & Menke, 1992).

CONTRIBUTING FACTORS

The traditional African American family structure has been described as an extended family in which most social, emotional and health needs were met. With the changing structure of the African American family and the diminishing support of the extended family, many more women have become vulnerable to becoming homeless. The dramatic increase of teen pregnancy among African American adolescents and laws that provide financial support for emancipated minors with children have enabled the rising homeless problem.

The adolescent while living independently, may no longer have the benefit of a consistent family support system, access to accurate information and guidance regarding child care, and household and financial management. This adolescent is at risk for becoming homeless. The increase of African American women with alcohol and/or substance abuse problems creates another at-risk group. They often lack problem-solving and management skills, a lack are further exacerbated by their substance use. These women, and particularly those with children, present with unique challenges and situations that require long term attention and multifaceted, wraparound services (L. Warkentin, personal interview, January 16, 2003).

Further, the dramatic increase of young African American males who are imprisoned, and those who experience an early death because of violence, has dramatically decreased possibilities of marriage for many young African American women, and specifically these young, sheltered homeless women. Additionally, this lack of eligible males has been exacerbated, by the rising number of upwardly mobile African American males who choose Caucasians or women of other nationalities as mates. Thus, for African American women in general, and particularly African American homeless women, the prospect of a stable home provided through marriage is considerably decreased (Billingsley, 1992, Chap. 1; Tucker & Mitchell-Kernan, 1995, Chap. 7).

Homeless women are confronted with multiple, simultaneous crises at a time when their self-esteem and coping mechanisms are significantly diminished. The precipitating causes of their homelessness may vary from family violence, family disputes, financial crises, substance use, conflicts with landlords resulting in evictions, fires, or many of the other contributing causes. Regardless of the multiplicity or gravity of those forces, commonalities exist in the experiences of homeless women.

ROLE OF AFRICAN AMERICAN WOMEN

Historically, the African American woman living in American society experiences many contradictions. During slavery, these women were intricately involved in the households of their slave masters. Many learned useful skills that provided opportunities for employment and in many situations, the African American woman was the primary breadwinner in the family, after slavery ended. At the same time, African American males were faced with more discrimination in social and employment situations, and thus could not fully assume the role of the head of the household. Thus, the strength of the African American woman was applauded and criticized at the same time. The applause came as many of these women overcame all odds to establish and maintain their homes and families. However, this situation tended to create female-dominated households, which to some extent, suppressed the role of the African American male. The overwhelming lack of authority and power felt by many African American males may eventually lead to out of marriage relationships and abandonment of their families by many of the men. In addition, African American women experience higher rates of intimate partner violence and homicide than white women (Lee et al., 2002). Subsequently, this dominant posture of many African American women has been repeatedly cited as the primary cause of many failed marriages.

WOMEN ON THE STREETS

During the last twenty years, the incarceration rate for African American women has tripled, and by 1995, one in every seven women arrested for a drug offense was sent to prison. In 2000, the Bureau of Justice Statistics documented that 83,668 women were imprisoned and 44 percent of that number were African American. During the period from 1986 to 1991, the number of African American women incarcerated in state prisons for a drug offense rose by 828 percent (Banks, 2003, pp. 44, 1; Elmore, 2004, p. 125). Of importance is that these women may be banned for life from receiving welfare benefits and from living in public housing and may lose access to student loans for higher education; however, these regulations vary state by state (Petersilia, 2003, Chap. 6; Elmore, 2004, p. 129). Many formerly incarcerated women become homeless as a result of these circumstances.

Other homeless women on the streets may include those with chronic mental illness, personality disorders, disaffiliation from a home base, or are on the streets as a result of eviction or rotation out of a shelter. If they are substance abusers suffering from some degree of mental illness, they may resist the admission policies and regulations of a traditional homeless shelter, or view the streets as a safer place than a shelter (Bachrach, 1987). Whatever the reason, women on the streets are more vulnerable to personal assaults and may become victims of crime and rape. The threat of violence for these women is ever present. Homeless women on the streets, particularly those who are drug dependent, precariously survive by using a street economy of sex work, shoplifting, and drug dealing (Epele, 2002). Epele describes how this reality becomes more profound by the female subordination promoted by the male-centered street ideology (2002).

This gender inequality and violence promote vulnerability of these women to HIV/AIDS. Local authorities in the Buffalo, New York area describe anecdotal data from these women who feel they use the men to achieve their own personal goals (L. Warkentin, personal interview, January 16, 2004). They are also at risk for health problems such as respiratory infections, skin disorders, and hypothermia in colder climates. Foot problems are rampant because many of these women walk for long distances with poor footgear. Other health problems such as varicose veins and chronic edema of the lower extremities are prevalent. These women may be resistant to accepting help from traditional health-related and social service systems, and rely primarily on the social network of individuals they develop for support.

WOMEN WITH CHILDREN IN SHELTERS

Homeless shelters were primarily established to address food and shelter needs of single homeless men, but they have undergone major changes with the dramatic increase of homeless women and families. More family-oriented shelters are available and many of them now provide health, financial, social, and other services. However, the structure, comprehensiveness, and continuity of the services provided in these shelters often falls short of the pressing needs of the recipients. While some model programs do exist, many others have experienced difficulties with client selection, program approaches, and inappropriate staffing mixes.

Many of this group of women and children reflect the negative consequences of social and economic trends that have severely affected the lives of the very poor. Financial, housing, educational, social, and family deficits placed them on a slippery slope from being very poor to homeless. These women have multiple crises in their lives as they move down the economic ladder and are unable to maintain a stable home and lifestyle. Family structure and cohesion particularly among teenage mothers may have never been established. The continuous burden of stress related to meeting basic survival needs and eventual transiency often leaves little time for nurturing their children.

As a result of this disruption and trauma, these women exhibit high levels of anxiety, uncertainty and chaos in their lives. Thus, it becomes difficult to function as a consistent and supportive parent. They must assume full responsibility for the children over a twenty-four-hour period in a homeless shelter and parent under less than desirable circumstances. The lack of affordable day care options and baby-sitting services within shelters may interfere with the satisfaction derived from motherhood; often experienced by nonsheltered mothers who have support systems, and parent under more desirable circumstances.

Mothers in these situations do not have an outlet for the release of tension, more common for unsheltered mothers. Because of the multiple and simultaneous issues with which they are dealing, the mother's attention span often is limited. As a result, it is difficult at times to provide constructive disciplinary boundaries for their children. The least deviation from perfection may spur some overzealous staff member to report the mother for child neglect or abuse. At times, the suspect behavior may simply represent cultural differences in child-rearing practices.

HEALTH OF HOMELESS WOMEN

The health status and health care of African Americans, has been significantly influenced by racial discrimination and racism in American society (Williams et al., 2003; Adams, 1995). Racial discrimination has limited the access of African Americans to higher incomes, improved health care, adequate housing, and education, all factors necessary to achieve modern levels of health and mortality (Thomas, 2001; Williams, 2002). Structural barriers exist that decrease access to health services and dealing with these structural barriers and negative racial behaviors of providers may increase stress-related health problems (Jackson et al., 2001; Alley et al., 1998; Hogue & Hargrave, 1993). African American homeless women are particularly vulnerable to these circumstances.

The data clearly demonstrate that homeless women generally manifest some common patterns of poor health that occur repeatedly (Luck et al., 2002; Nayamathi et al., 2000; Gelberg et al., 1997; Bassuk et al., 1996; Lim et al., 2002). Toothaches, caries, and draining and damaged teeth are almost the norm, secondary to battering, poor oral hygiene, and last-resort dental care, which generally ends up in multiple extractions. Gynecological problems related to sexual abuse, sexually transmitted disease, and inadequate care are common. Pregnant women often do not receive prenatal care (Wenzel et al., 2001; Wright et al., 1998, Chap. 8). Other common occurring problems include depression, nutritional deficiencies, infestations, alcohol and drug abuse, and social isolation, to name a few (Amarasingham et al., 2001; Breakey et al., 1989; Burt & Cohen, 1989; Ugarriza & Fallon, 1994). A lack of coordinated, regular medical, dental, and prenatal care is most often determined to precede these health problems (Han et al., 2003; Adkins & Fields, 1992). These women are often in need of mental health services, particularly those who have been victims of domestic violence.

In an overview of the literature of the mental health problems of homeless women, it was found that homeless women exhibited disproportionately high rates of mental disorders. Nonwhite women were only half as likely to receive inpatient care or outpatient psychiatric treatment. More nonwhites had desired but not obtained psychiatric treatment. The authors concluded that many homeless women with serious mental health problems were not receiving needed care, due in part to the lack of perception of a mental health problem and the lack of services designed to meet the special needs of homeless women (Robertson & Winkleby, 1996). Furthermore, data confirmed that homeless single women have higher rates of psychiatric disorders than homeless men (Buckner et al., 1993).

Of particular concern is the risk of homeless women and particularly African American women for several potential life-threatening diseases. Startling trends have recently been reported, related to the spread of HIV/AIDS. Currently, racial and ethnic populations account for 25 percent of the total U.S. population; however, they represent more than 50 percent of the cumulative U.S. AIDS cases (Needle et al., 2003). By 1998, 65 percent of the newly reported AIDS cases were among Black and Hispanic adults. Since 1999, death rates have declined markedly, but the decline was smallest among African American women and death rates were the highest among African American women when compared to whites (U.S. Census Bureau, 1998; Centers for Disease Control and Prevention [CDC], 1999; Karon et al., 2001). In a study of homeless women of reproductive age, 64 percent had engaged in unprotected sex and 22 percent had traded sex for other commodities (Kilbourne et al., 2002).

Homeless women, in general, are at greater risk for infection due to engaging in prostitution and other high-risk behaviors. Many of them have been raped, are reported intravenous drug users, or diagnosed as mentally ill. They represent a very endangered group. HIV testing may be done, yet the woman may have left the shelter before the results were given to her. In a recent survey, it was found that many women did not follow up for gynecological care because they forgot their appointments. Also, they did not want to leave the safe environment of the shelter to keep outside appointments (Johnstone et al., 1993). The upsurge of tuberculosis after many years of decline is believed to be related to the HIV epidemic. Persons who have compromised immune systems by HIV are much more susceptible to developing tuberculosis (Han et al., 2003; Colson et al., 1994).

The health status of African American homeless women continues to be an issue. Historically, African Americans were denied health care because of segregation and discrimination. An extensive folk medicine practice was utilized by many African Americans, in part, a response to the lack of access to adequate medical and health care. Today, many of the access barriers have been removed. However, many African Americans still receive less than adequate health care,

are disproportionately cared for in hospital clinics, and have poorer health care outcomes. African Americans continue to experience higher rates of chronic diseases, such as cancer, heart disease, and strokes, and live an average five years less than Caucasians (Ibrahim et al., 2003; Smedley et al., 2003). As a group, they tend to ignore symptoms until they become intolerable, and thus are more often diagnosed when diseases have already caused permanent damage.

African American women have higher rates of infant death, diabetes mellitus, breast cancer, hysterectomies, and tubal ligations. While a significant number of African American women are obese, their nutritional status is often below average. Dietary patterns that are culturally determined contribute to this problem and are difficult to change. In addition, many African American women, and particularly homeless women, have very little knowledge or accurate information about their own bodies. Generally, these women lack knowledge of health maintenance and health promotion approaches (Adkins & Fields, 1992).

HEALTH OF HOMELESS CHILDREN

A survey of 25 U.S. cities found that families with children accounted for 40 percent of the homeless population (U.S. Conference of Mayors, 2003) who are homeless on average of 10 months at a time (U.S. Department of Health and Human Services [DHHS], 2001). Moreover 85 percent of homeless children are headed by single mothers and 41 percent of these children are aged one to five (Redlener, 1999; Better Homes Fund, 1999). By all measurement of current trends, this phenomenon will continue to increase.

Domestic violence contributes to homelessness among families. Children from these families experience emotional and psychological effects from the fear and insecurity of living in these circumstances (NCH, 2001; Bassuk et al., 1997). The issues of homeless children are further compounded by their transiency, the emotional and psychological effects of violence, living in a shelter, and lack of consistent patterns of seeking health care (Percy, 1995; Baumann, 1993). Extreme poverty and housing instability are particularly harmful during the earliest years of childhood. Few studies have examined the long term-effects of homelessness on the children who share a nomadic lifestyle with their mothers. The chaotic circumstances of their lives is often displayed in the behavior of the children (Hausman & Hammen, 1993). Acting-out behavior, such as regression to bed wetting and other earlier behaviors, and temper tantrums are not uncommon.

Homeless children have disproportionately high levels of poor academic skills, erratic school attendance, and school failure. School-aged homeless children face barriers to enrolling and attending school, including transportation problems, residency requirements, inability to obtain previous school records, and lack of clothing and school supplies. Developmental screening has identified more developmental lags in homeless pre-school children than among school-age children, and academic problems are common (Page et al., 1993; Bassuk & Rosenberg, 1990). It has been noted that homeless children face many barriers to educational services primarily due to their mobility and subsequent poor transfer of records. In a study of homeless children in Los Angeles, California, it was found that almost half of the children merited a special education evaluation, yet less than one-quarter of those with a disability had ever received special education testing or enrolled in special classes (Zima, 1997).

Homelessness is an important risk factor for a number of health issues that affect homeless children. Data remains limited; however, the available data suggest an overall increased morbidity among homeless children. Homeless parents more often rate their children's health as only fair or poor (Weinreb et al., 1998; Menke & Wagner, 1997). Homeless parents generally do not perceive their children as healthy, they often have multiple health problems and are more likely to be seen in the emergency room (Weinreb et al., 1998; Berti et al., 2001; Bassuk et al., 1996; Bassuk et al., 1997; Hatton, 1997; Redlener, 1999).

Homeless families often live in crowded quarters that increase the risk of common infectious diseases of childhood such as upper respiratory infections, ear infections and diarrhea (Murata et al., 1992; Children's Health Fund, 1999). Homeless children often have multiple health problems and have higher rates of asthma, ear infections, stomach problems and speech problems (Better Homes Fund, 1990; Berti et al., 2001). Poor housing and negative environmental surroundings further expose homeless children to risk of injury and lead toxicity (DHHS, 2001). For homeless children, access to nutritious food is problematic. Thus, chronic malnutrition may lead to lack of attainment of normal height, dental caries and vision problems (Fierman et al., 1991; Page et al., 1993; Baumann, 1996).

ISSUES OF PROVIDING CARE

Given the current situation of the health status of African Americans, the challenge of providing health care and appropriate follow-up for homeless women is a major one. In general, they do not seek health care in a timely manner. Often, other women or shelter staff must encourage the client to go to the health clinic. This reluctance is due to several factors. First, because they have so many pressing concerns in the shelter such as applying for public benefits, looking for housing, seeking employment, and so on, health care is not an immediate priority. Second, many of these women have had negative experiences with other health care providers, and particularly with white male physicians. And third, most of the women do not have health insurance, and paying for care is a major barrier. Health care services when provided free of charge in homeless shelters are not without problems. Providers attest to difficulties with client's seeking health care, follow-up, and continuity of care.

Health services that are provided in a shelter generally address episodic health problems amenable to uncomplicated interventions and treatments. The women often refuse to accept referrals to other clinics and hospitals, due to possible embarrassment about their current homeless situation, long waits, inability to pay for services, and negative attitudes of health care professionals.

A recent study completed in the city of Buffalo, New York, by the UB Center for Urban Studies and the UB Center for Research in Primary Care (2001) examined the health, social, economic, cultural, and lifestyle issues that affect the health status of a primarily African American, poor, urban community. The findings are consistent with the issues facing the homeless who are in need of health care. Access to health care and on overuse of emergency rooms for primary care, inability to pay for prescriptions and other treatments, difficulty communicating or establishing rapport with health professionals and lack of preventative care were among the key findings. Of note was the fact that while 80 percent of these inner city respondents had some form of health insurance, other barriers of getting time off from work to visit a physician and obtaining child care were mentioned. It is important to note that similar barriers in obtaining health care services are often experienced by the homeless client, yet no segment of this population was acknowledged or mentioned in that report.

ISSUES OF POWERLESSNESS

Life in a shelter is stressful and crisis prone. Women enter the shelter environment dealing with a series of dramatic and traumatic events in their lives. Within this environment they lose further control over their lives. Adult women are required to live in cramped quarters, share meals with total strangers, and face a bureaucratic system that is not always user friendly. Mandates are often imposed on them without benefit of a complete assessment of their needs. What these women need, first and foremost, is acceptance and nonjudgmental understanding. Women in the shelter often make reference to the lack of sensitivity of staff, as they are pushed to apply for social services and make contacts with housing agencies. Shelter staff may be inexperienced, nonprofessional, and lack cultural awareness and sensitivity. These staff may have limited skills and inadequate training to assist women in emotional crisis or those in need of immediate psychiatric help.

Currently, the Buffalo, New York, Cornerstone Manor, houses up to sixty homeless women and children on a daily basis. Over 60 percent of the women in this particular shelter are admitted with no health insurance due to their transiency and lack of follow up of previous applications. Several initiatives undertaken by the shelter administration have transformed Cornerstone Manor into a comprehensive, long-term, life-changing program for the residents. The staff work with the women to identify the causes of their homelessness and then challenge and empower the women to make changes in their lives. Cornerstone Manor provides in-house education and job training, addiction recovery programs, a free pediatric and adult clinic and preventative health care. The work of Hodnicki and Horner (1993) supports this model.

This approach of one homeless shelter addresses the reality that the array of social and psychological services previously available to communities through public programs, have been severely curtailed or eliminated. Thus, this not for profit, nondenominational, religious organization has replaced the "Safety Net," no longer in existence through public funds in this particular community.

The Nursing Center for the Homeless in Buffalo, New York, previously identified this need and provided the foundation for the current program at

Cornerstone Manor in Buffalo, New York (DHHS, 1993). The Nursing Center demonstrated the need to address the health care problems of the homeless in an holistic model with special attention to their emotional and psychological needs, through advocacy and the use of support groups.

RECOMMENDATIONS

It has been noted that persistent racial disparities in health access, quality and status reflect a health care system that is not equally responsive to the needs of a racially and ethnically diverse female population (Jackson et al., 2001). New models of care are needed particularly for African American homeless women. There is a critical need for more comprehensive, culturally sensitive health and supportive services provided in safe surroundings for these women and their children.

For the many women, who become homeless as a result of a combination of factors including drug and alcohol abuse, leaving the shelter without a comprehensive plan of services simply predisposes them to homelessness in the future. The combination of homelessness, mental illness and substance abuse creates a self-perpetuating cycle that is difficult to interrupt (Drury, 2003). More residential programs and quality housing are needed to provide these women with opportunities to acquire work and parenting skills, and increase self-esteem. The referral to transitional housing provides a longer training time and a better opportunity to address their lack of skills and then move to permanent housing. Follow-up is needed after the women leave the shelter, to reinforce new behaviors, and to prevent homelessness in the future (Kinzel, 1993). Case managers have been effective in assisting these women to address the complex eligibility criteria and application procedures for important programs available to them (Heslin et al., 2003).

The work of Montgomery (1994) is supportive of these findings. She conducted a preliminary investigation of homeless women to determine how they overcame their circumstances. Most of the women had been physically or sexually abused as children. Others had been neglected or abandoned by their mothers. The respondents viewed their homelessness as a temporary disruption that occurred when they attempted to change their circumstances and move on to a better life. The personal strengths that the women identified were: a stubborn sense of pride, positive orientation, moral structure, and a clarity of focus that grew out of the first three qualities. Connection with a larger community helped these women to mobilize their strengths and rebuild their lives (Montgomery, 1994). Several studies have documented the influence of social support in determining how and when homeless persons utilize available services (Luck et al., 2002; Hatton, 2001; Nyamathi et al., 2000; Fitzpatrick et al., 2003).

Those individuals who work with African American homeless women should be oriented to the special emotional and psychosocial needs of this group. Providers should be sensitive to issues of race and how this relates to their homelessness. They also need to be sensitive to the unique position of a homeless person and the related stress that threatens an individual's sense of

mastery and confidence (Baumann, 1993). The loss of self-esteem, powerlessness, and victimization among these women must be addressed in order to
empower them to take control of their lives. Those women that are unable to set
directions and develop goals or plans for "getting on with their lives," are prone
to experience homelessness over a long-term period. Racial discrimination
continues to exist in the job and housing markets, in bureaucratic agency policies and in attitudes of providers and these factors impede their progress toward
financial independence. Each of these factors must be addressed with understanding and positive, culturally relevant concern, if help is to be given to these
clients.

SUMMARY AND CONCLUSIONS

The homeless problem in contemporary society and specifically the United
States, has been created in part by political, economic, and societal forces that
have included drastic and severe federal funding cuts in affordable housing and
financial assistance for low-income individuals. Further, the current economic
downturn, technological changes and globalization of the workplace continues
to disproportionately affect those most economically disadvantaged. The lasting
effect of these changes is a decline of unskilled, and low-paying jobs for these
groups and a lack of specific preparation for the positions that are available. At
the same time, the stock of safe, affordable housing in urban areas has been
reduced (Erie County Commission on Homelessness, personal interview, January 2004).

There are many pathways to homelessness; most include individual, family,
and economic factors. According to one author, "Homelessness is not a characteristic of people, but rather a condition in which some people find themselves
at some point and time" (Blasi, 1990). The health, social, and housing needs of
homeless women are great and the available services generally, do not meet their
identified needs. The increased numbers of African American homeless women
with children is a group that is particularly vulnerable to permanent homelessness and its consequences.

In spite of the increasing numbers of homeless women with children, there is
no national or organized program to address the multiple issues faced by these
homeless women. There is no public outcry for addressing the root causes of
homelessness. Current programs do not effectively address the complex and
long-term problems of this group. The existing federal legislation, Public
Law 100-77 (Stewart B. McKinney Act of 1987), authorized funding for emergency shelters and a variety of programs. This legislation does not provide
for development of low-rent housing or adequate incomes for extremely poor
people.

The literature review conducted since 1995 clearly indicates that the situation
has worsened. Policymakers and public officials should recognize the effects of
homelessness on individuals and families. The psychological effects and the
disruption of normal parenting are cause enough for action. Without attention,
all indications are that this problem will threaten the physical and mental health

of the next generation of American citizens, and particularly those who are African American.

To date, concerted government support of programs to assist the homeless has been lacking. What is needed is a program of antipoverty policies and affordable housing. At a time when elected officials are forging ahead with a mandate to eliminate government control, a federal initiative is needed to coordinate resources and provide leadership to states to encourage a pro-active approach to a contemporary problem that will undoubtedly increase. The lack of health care to this group will present an ever-increasing public health problem for the majority society. The alternative will be an ever-increasing number of citizens, and especially children, who will be ill prepared to compete in the twenty-first century. The African American community, and particularly the churches, should provide the leadership in development of effective, realistic, and coordinated efforts of all major service and public housing agencies to address this crisis.

REFERENCES

Adams, D. L. 1995. *Health Issues for Women of Color*. Thousand Oaks, CA: Sage Publications.

Adkins, C. B., and J. Fields. 1992. "Health Care Values of Homeless Women and Their Children." *Family Community Health*, 15(3):20–29.

Alley, N., C. Macnee, S. Aurora, and A. Alley. 1998. "Health Promotion Lifestyles of Women Experiencing Crises." *Journal of Community Health Nursing*, 15(2):91–99.

Amarasingham, R., S. H. Spalding, and R. J. Anderson. 2001. "Disease Conditions Most Frequently Evaluated among the Homeless in Dallas." *Health Care for the Poor and Underserved*, 12(2):162–176.

Bachrach, L. L. 1987. "Homeless Women: A Context for Health Planning." *The Milbank Quarterly*, 65(3):371–396.

Banks, C. 2003. *Women in Prison*. Santa Barbara, CA: ABC-CLIO.

Bassuk, E. L. 1993. "Social and Economic Hardships of Homeless and Other Poor Women." *American Journal of Orthopsychiatry*, 63(3):340–347.

Bassuk, E. L., A. Browne, and J. C. Buckner. 1996. "Single Mothers and Welfare." *Scientific American*, 275(4):60–67.

Bassuk, E. L., L. Weinreb, J. C. Buckner, A. Browne, A. Salomon, and S. S. Bassuk. 1996. "The Characteristics and Needs of Sheltered and Low Income Housed Mothers." *Journal of the American Medical Association*, 276, 640–646.

Bassuk, E. L., L. F. Weinreb, R. Dawson, J. N. Perloff, and J. C. Buckner. 1997. "Determinants of Behavior in Homeless and Low-income Housed Preschool Children." *Pediatrics*, 100, 92–100.

Bassuk, E. L., and L. Rosenberg. 1990. "Psychosocial Characteristics of Homeless Children and Children with Homes." *Pediatrics*, 85, 257–261.

Baumann, G. L. 1993. "The Meaning of Being Homeless." *Scholarly Inquiry for Nursing Practice: An International Journal*, 7(1):59–70.

Baumann, S. L. 1996. "Feeling Uncomfortable: Children in Families with No Place of Their Own." *Nursing Science Quarterly*, 9(4):152–159.

Berti, L. C., S. Zylbert, and L. Rolnitzky. 2001. "Comparison of Health Statures of Children Using a School-based Health Centers for Comprehensive Care." *Journal of Pediatric Health Care*, 15, 244–250.

The Better Homes Fund. 1999. *Homeless Children: America's New Outcasts*. Newton, MA: Author.

Billingsley, A. 1992. *Climbing Jacob's Ladder* (Chap. 11). New York, London: Simon & Schuster.

Blasi, G. L. 1990. "Social Policy and Social Science Research on Homelessness." *Journal of Social Issues*, 46(4):207–219.

Breakey, W. M. 1997. "Editorial: It's Time for the Public Health Community to Declare War on Homelessness." *American Journal of Public Health*, 87(2):153–154.

Breakey, W. M., P. J. Fischer, M. Kramer, G. Nestadt, A. J. Romanoski, A. Ross, R. M. Royall, and O. C. Stine. 1989. "Health and Mental Health Problems of Homeless Men and Women in Baltimore." *Journal of the American Medical Association*, 262(10):1352–1357.

Browne, A. 1993. "Family Violence and Homelessness: The Relevance of Trauma Histories in the Lives of Homeless Women." *American Journal of Orthopsychiatry*, 63(3):370–384.

Buckner, J. C., E. L. Bassuk, and B. T. Zima. 1993. "Mental Health Issues Affecting Homeless Women." *American Journal Orthopsychiatry*, 63(3):385.

Burg, M. A. 1994. "Health Problems of Sheltered Homeless Women and Their Dependent Children." *Health and Social Work*, 19, 125–131.

Burt, M. R., and B. E. Cohen. 1989. "Differences among Homeless Single Women, Women with Children, and Single Men." *Social Problems*, 36(5):508–524.

Centers for Disease Control & Prevention. 1995. "Update: AIDS among Women—United States, 1994." *Morbidity and Mortality Weekly Report*, 44(5):8184.

———. 1999. *HIV Surveillance Report*, 11, no. 1.

Colson, P., E. Susser, and E. Valencia. 1994. "HIV and TB among People Who Are Homeless and Mentally Ill." *Psychosocial Rehabilitation Journal*, 17(4):157–159.

Division of Nursing. 1993. Special Project Grants Program in the Nursing Education Practice Resources Branch, Division of Nursing, U.S. Department of Health and Human Services, Public Health Service, Health Resources and Services Administration, Bureau of Health Professions Administration. Grant #5D106000305 and Grant #2D 106003-04.

Drury, L. J. 2003. "Community Care for People Who Are Homeless and Mentally Ill." *Journal of Health Care for the Poor and Underserved*, 14(2):194–207.

Elmore, J. V. 2004. *Fighting for Your Life*. Phoenix, AZ: Amber Books.

Epele, M. E. 2002. "Gender, Violence and HIV: Women's Survival in the Streets." *Culture, Medicine and Psychiatry*, 26(1):33–54.

Erie County Commission On Homelessness. 2003. *Understanding Homelessness: A Report To the Community*. Buffalo, NY: Author.

Fierman, A. H., B. P. Dreyer, P. J. Acker, and L. Legano. 1993. "Status of Immunization and Iron Nutrition in New York City Homeless Children." *Clinical Pediatrics*, 32, 151–155.

Fitzpatrick, K. M., M. E. LaGory, and F. J. Ritchey. 2003. "Factors Associated with Health-compromising Behaviors among the Homeless." *Journal of Health Care for the Poor and Underserved*, 14(1):70–86.

Gelberg, L., T. C. Gallagher, R. M. Andersen, and P. Koegel. 1997. "Competing Priorities as a Barrier to Medical Care among Homeless Adults in Los Angeles." *American Journal of Public Health*, 87, 217–220.

Goering, P., D. Paduchak, and J. Durbin. 1990. "Housing Homeless Women: A Consumer Preference Study." *Housing and Community Psychiatry*, 41(6):790–794.

Han, B., B. L. Wells, and A. M. Taylor. 2003. "Use of the Homeless Program Services and Other Health Care Services by Homeless Adults." *Journal of Health Care for the Poor and Underserved,* 14(1):87–99.

Hatchett, S., J. Veroff, and E. Douvan. 1995. "Marital Instability among Black and White Couples in Early Marriage." In M. B. Tucker and C. Mitchell-Kernan (Eds.), *The Decline in Marriage among African Americans* (Chap. 7). New York: Russell Sage Foundation.

Hatton, D. 1997. "Managing Health Problems among Homeless Women with Children in a Transitional Shelter." *Image: Journal of Nursing Scholarship,* 29(1):3–37.

Hatton, D. C. 2001. "Homeless Women's Access to Health Services: A Study of Social Networks and Managed Care in the U.S." *Women and Health,* 33(4):149–161.

Hatton, D. C., D. Kleffel, S. Bennett, and E.A.N. Gaffrey. 2001. "Homeless Women and Children's Access to Health Care: A Paradox." *Journal of Community Health Nursing,* 18(1):25–34.

Hausman, B., and C. Hammen. 1993. "Parenting in Homeless Families: The Double Crisis." *American Journal of Orthopsychiatry,* 63(3):358–369.

Heslin, K.C., R.M. Anderson, and L. Gelberg. 2003. "Case Management and Access to Service for Homeless Women." *Journal of Health Care for the Poor and Underserved,* 14(1):34–51.

Hodnicki, R., and S. D. Horner. 1993. "Homeless Mothers Caring for Children in a Shelter." *Issues in Mental Health Nursing,* 14, 349–356.

Hogue, C.J., and M.A. Hargrave. 1993. "Class, Race and Infant Mortality in the United States." *American Journal of Public Health,* 83(1):9–12.

Hombs, M. E. 2001. *American Homelessness.* Santa Barbara, CA: ABC-CLIO.

Hopper, K., E. Susser, and S. Conover. 1985. "Economics of Makeshift: Deindustrialization and Homelessness in New York City." *Urban Anthropology,* 14, 183–235.

Hunter, J. K. 1995. "Homelessness: Nursing Care for a Vulnerable Population." *Journal of the New York State Nurses Association,* 26(1):37–39.

Ibrahim, S. A., S. B. Thomas, and M. J. Fine. 2003. "Achieving Health Equity: An Incremental Journal" [Editorial]. *American Journal of Public Health,* 93(10): 1619–1621.

"The Institute for Children and Poverty." 1991. *Homes for the Homeless.* New York: Author.

Interagency Council on the Homeless. 1991. *The 1990 Annual Report of the Interagency Council on the Homeless.* Washington, DC: Author.

Jackson, S., D. Camacho, K. M. Freund, J. A. Bigby, J. Walcott-McQuigg, E. Hughes, A. Nunez, W. Dillard, C. Weiner, T. Weitz, and A. Zerr. 2001. "Women's Health Centers and Minority Women: Addressing Barriers to Care." The National Centers of Excellence in Women's Health. *Journal of Women's Health and Gender-Based Medicines,* 10(6):551–559.

Johnstone, H., M. Tornabene, and J. Marcinak. 1993. "Incidence of Sexually Transmitted Diseases and Pap Smear Results in Female Homeless Clients from the Chicago Outreach Project." *Health Care for Women International,* 14, 293–299.

Karon, J. M., P. L. Fleming, R. W. Stekater, and K. M. De Cock. 2001. "HIV in the United States at the Turn of the Century: An Epidemic in Transition." *American Journal of Public Health,* 91(7):1060–1068.

Kemsley, M., and J. K. Hunter. 1992. "Homeless Children and Families: Clinical Research Issues." *Issues in Comprehensive Pediatric Nursing,* 16, 99–108.

Kilbourne, A. M., B. Herndon, R. M. Andersen, S. L. Wenzel, and L. Gelberg. 2002. "Psychiatric Symptoms, Health Services, and HIV Risk Factors among Homeless Women." *Journal of Health Care for the Poor and Underserved,* 13(1):49–65.

Kinzel, D. M. 1993. "Response to the Meaning of Being Homeless?" *Scholarly Inquiry for Nursing Practice: An International Journal,* 7(1):71–73.

Lee, R. N., V. L. Sanders-Thompson, and M. B. Mechanic. 2002. Intimate Partner Violence and Women of Color: A Call for Innovations." *American Journal of Public Health,* 92(4):530–534.

Lim, Y. W., R. Andersen, B. Leake, W. Cunningham, and L. Gelberg. 2002. "How Accessible Is Medical Care for Homeless Women?" *Medical Care,* 40(6):510–520.

Luck, J., R. Andersen, S. Wenzel, L. Arangua, D. Wood, and L. Gelberg. 2002. "Providers of Primary Care to Homeless Women in Los Angeles County." *Journal of Ambulatory Care Management,* 25(2):53–67.

Lyon-Callo, V. 2000. "Medicalizing Homelessness: The Production of Self-blame and Self-governing within Homeless Shelters." *Medical Anthropology Quarterly,* 14(3):328–345.

Marcuse, P. 1989. "Gentrification, Homelessness, and the Work Process." *Housing Studies,* 4, 211–220.

Menke, E. M., and J. D. Wagner. 1997. "A Comparative Study of Homeless, Previously Homeless, and Never Homeless School-aged Children's Health." *Issues in Comprehensive Pediatric Nursing,* 20, 153–173.

Montgomery, C. 1994. "Swimming Upstream: The Strengths of Women Who Survive Homelessness." *Advances in Nursing Science,* 16(3):34–45.

Murata, J., J. P. Mace, A. Strehlow, and P. Sheuler. 1992. "Disease Patterns in Homeless Children: A Comparison with National Data." *Journal of Pediatric Nursing,* 7, 196–204.

Myrdal, G. 1944. *An American Dilemma.* New York: Harper & Bros.

National Coalition for the Homeless. 2001. *Homeless Families with Children.* NCH Fact Sheet #7. Washington, DC: National Coalition for the Homeless.

Needle, R. H., M. Trotter Singer, C. Bates, B. Page, D. Metzger, and L. H. Marcelin. 2003. "Rapid Assessment of the HIV/AIDS Crisis in Racial and Ethnic Minority Communities: An Approach for Timely Community Interventions." *American Journal of Public Health,* 93(6):970–979.

Nyamathi, A., B. Leake, C. Keenan, and L. Galberg. 2000. "Type of Social Support among Homeless Women: Its Impact on Psychosocial Resources, Health and Health Behaviors, and Use of Health Services." *Nursing Research,* 49(6):318–326.

Page, A. J., A. D. Ainsworth, and M. A. Pett. 1993. "Homeless Families and Their Children's Health Problems: A Utah Urban Experience." *Western Journal of Medicine,* 158, 30–35.

Percy, M. S. 1995. "Children from Homeless Families Describe What Is Special in Their Lives." *Holistic Nursing Practice,* 9(4):24–33.

Petersilia, J. 2003. *When Prisoners Come Home.* Oxford, New York: Oxford University Press.

Prentice, B. 1993. "Homelessness and Public Policy." In J. Hunter, (Ed.), *Nursing and Health Care for the Homeless* (pp. 17–28). Albany: State University of New York Press.

Public Law 100-77. 1987. Stewart B. McKinney Act of 1987.

Redlener, S. 1999. *Still in Crisis: The Health Status of New York's Homeless Children.* New York: The Children's Health Fund.

Robertson, N. J., and M. A. Winkleby. 1996. "Mental Health Problems of Homeless Women and Differences across Subgroups." *Annual Review of Public Health,* 17, 311–336.

Rossi, P. 1989. *Without Shelter* (Chap. 1). New York: Priority Press Publications.

Skelly, A. H., M. Kemsley, J. K. Hunter, C. Getty, and J. Shipman. 1990. "A Survey of Health Perceptions of the Homeless." *Journal of the New York State Nurses Association,* 21(2):20–24.

Smedley, B. D., A. Y. Stith, and A. R. Nelson. 2003. *Unequal Treatment Confronting Racial and Ethnic Disparities in Health Care.* Institute of Medicine. Washington, DC: National Academies Press.

Thomas, S. B. 2001. "The Color Line: Race Matters in the Elimination of Health Disparities." *American Journal of Public Health,* 91(7):1046–1047.

Tucker, M. B., and C. Mitchell-Kernan. 1995. *The Decline of Marriage among African-Americans: Causes, Consequences and Policy Implications.* New York: Russell Sage Foundation.

UB Center for Urban Studies, UB Center for Research in Primary Care and the Black Leadership Forum. 2001. *The Health Status of the Near East Side Black Community.* Funded by Kaleida Health, Buffalo, New York.

Ugarriza, D. N., and T. Fallon. 1994. "Nurses' Attitudes Toward Homeless Women: A Barrier to Change." *Nursing Outlook,* 42(1):26–29.

U.S. Census Bureau. 1998. *Statistical Abstract of the United States* (118th ed.). Washington, DC: U.S. Census Bureau.

U. S. Conference of Mayors. 1997. *A Status Report on Hunger and Homelessness in America's Cities: A 29-city Survey.* Washington, DC.

———. 2001. *A Status Report on Hunger and Homelessness in America's Cities: A 27-city Survey.* Washington, DC.

———. 2003. Hunger and Homelessness Survey. Washington, DC.

U.S. Department of Health and Human Services. Office of Disease Prevention and Health Promotion. 2001. *Healthy People 2010: Understanding and Improving Health.* Washington, DC: Author.

Wagner, J. D., and E. M. Menke. 1992. "Case Management of Homeless Families." *Clinical Nurse Specialist,* 6(2):65–71.

Weinreb, L., and J. C. Buckner. 1998. "Homeless Families: Program Responses and Public Policies." *American Journal of Orthopsychiatry,* 63(3):400–409.

Weinreb, L., R. Goldberg, E. L. Bassuk, and J. Perloff. 1998. "Determinants of Health and Service Use Patterns in Homeless and Low-income Housed Children." *Pediatrics,* 102, 554–562.

Wenzel, S. L., R. M. Andersen, D. S. Gifford, and L. Gelberg. 2001. "Homeless Women's Gynecological Symptoms and Use of Medical Care." *Health Care for the Poor and Underserved,* 12(3):323–341.

Williams, B. 1996. "There Goes the Neighborhood: Gentrification, Displacement, and Homelessness in Washington, DC. In Anna Lou Dehavenon (Ed.), *There's No Place Like Home: Anthropological Perspectives on Housing and Homelessness in the United States* (pp. 145–163). Westport, CT: Bergin & Garvey.

Williams, D. R. 2002. "Racial/Ethnic Variations in Women's Health: the Social Embeddedness of Health." *American Journal of Public Health,* 92(4):588–597.

Williams, D. R., H. W. Neighbors, and J. S. Jackson. 2003. "Racial/ethnic Discrimination and Health: Findings from Community Studies." *American Journal of Public Health,* 98(2):200–214.

Wingel, S. L., B. D. Leake, and L. Gelberg. 2000. "Health of Homeless Women with Recent Experience of Rape." *General Internal Medicine,* 15(4):265–268.

Wright, J. D., B. A. Rubin, and A. Joel. 1998. *Beside the Golden Door.* New York: Aldine De Gruyter.

Wright, T. 1997. *Out of Place*. Albany, NY: State University of New York Press.

Zima, B. T. 1997. "Sheltered Homeless Children: Their Eligibility and Unmet Need for Special Education Evaluations." *American Journal of Public Health*, 87(2): 236–240.

11

Informed Decisions: Paving the Way to Informed Consent

RHEA J. SIMMONS

"I am sorry, but you need to make a decision..."
These words underscore the importance of having the necessary informa-
tion to adequately respond and ultimately offer informed consent.

Do these words sound familiar? For some of us, these words resonate back to a time when we may have felt vulnerable while personally facing a health crisis, an acute illness or chronic condition, or they may represent an emotional period when a loved one was confronted with a serious health matter. Whatever the case, these words may have elicited feelings of anxiety, shock, fear, confusion, stress, or even denial. Ten relatively simple words have the power to render us emotionally crippled and remind us of our fragility and mortality. These words underscore the importance of having the necessary information to adequately respond and ultimately offer informed consent. Therefore, we need to pause and reflect on how we conceptualize decision making and the informed consent process during these critical periods in our lives.

In the matriarchal African American family, women make decisions about serious issues on a daily basis that have the potential to alter one's entire course of life. For example, women make decisions about challenges in life ranging from economics to medical care for ailing parents, education of children, catastrophic illness, counseling, custody, surgery, mental health treatment, and what constitutes good health care. In general, decisions about health and health problems are complex and frightening for everyone, regardless of age or gender. However, making a decision regarding a health matter may be one of the most daunting experiences in life. Fundamental to the decision making process is the responsibility of giving consent for services or treatment, while oftentimes making these decisions based on rather limited information.

Statistics on illness and disease among African American women reflect disparities in health status and disproportions in incidence and prevalence, as compared to other population groups (Finkelstein et al., 2004; Pikler & Winterowd, 2003; Stover et al., 2001). Cardiovascular disease, stroke, hypertension, diabetes, and cancer are among those that African American women need to be particularly aware of due to ethnicity, as well as personal and family history. Discussion of these illnesses and diseases is deferred to other chapters in this book. However, this chapter serves to focus attention on the importance of making informed decisions necessary for giving informed consent for everyday health and related health care matters.

Informed consent is a phrase that is generally associated with research or clinical trials in medicine. More specifically, informed consent is central to discussions about human subject research. From a historical perspective, contemporary concern about ethical research practices and informed consent dates back to 1947 with the establishment of the Universal Declaration of Human Rights (Annas, 1998) and the 1979 "Belmont Report," *Ethical Guidelines for the Protection of Human Subjects in Research* (National Commission for the Protection of Human Subjects of Biomedical and Behavioral Research, 1979; Nelson-Marten & Rich, 1999). Despite these protections, there are a number of documented cases of significant research abuse of human subjects and ethical misconduct. Among the most widely known cases of abusive treatment of human research participants is the 1932 Tuskegee Syphilis Study of untreated syphilis in Black males that was conducted by the U.S. Public Health Service (Freimuth et al., 2001). Another case illustrating misconduct and lack of informed consent in human research is the Goldzieher Oral Contraceptives Study of Mexican American Women (Goldzieher et al., 1971), which contributed to women being designated as a vulnerable population category in human subject research by the Department of Health and Human Services.

Federal guidelines have been reemphasized to address and provide for the ethical treatment of human subjects in research (U.S. Department of Health and Human Services, 1991), and professional associations have established standards to provide safeguards for the use and treatment of human participants in research. Institutional Review Boards (IRBs) have been established to review research protocols as a means to ensure the ethical treatment of participants in research. To briefly summarize, major conditions of informed consent refer to subjects or participants of research having specific and understandable information including purpose of study and duration, voluntary participation, opportunities to decline from participation, risks and benefits, alternative treatments or procedures, confidentiality, compensation, and persons available for additional information.

On a daily basis, informed consent relative to patients and their health should be protected just like "human subjects in research." Parallel safeguards and guidelines for informed consent are in existence for health care providers. For example, the American Medical Association (1997) has a published code of ethics for medical practitioners that addresses informed consent. The American Psychological Association (2002) has delineated ethical principles for psychologists and a code of conduct, which also includes requirements for informed consent. The American College of Obstetricians and Gynecologists (1989) has also articulated "elements of informed consent" that must be discussed between patient and physician.

However, the real question is, *"Do we exercise informed consent in our everyday decisions about health and health care related issues?"* For instance, when you give consent for a medical procedure or agree to a service or treatment recommended by your physician, are you *really* cognizant of the benefits and potential harms? If you are taking medication for a health problem, are you comfortable with your level of understanding about the contraindications? Recognizing that overall health is enhanced our emotional, spiritual, psychological, and social well-being, and dependent on our understanding of diet, exercise, nutrition, daily health practices, lifestyle, and health history (both individual and familial), what can we do to ensure that we make the best decisions possible to protect and preserve our health? We can make informed decisions about our health by engaging in informed consent. Informed consent is a process predicated on informed decisions. The two are intertwined and should be considered as dependent on each other.

The health care field represents one of the best illustrations of the relationship between informed decisions and the informed consent process. For example, research has shown that African American women have particular concerns about health and the potential for diseases. Wilcox et al. (2002) examined health concerns, illness, and diseases among women aged 36–91 and found that African American and Native American women were more worried about developing cancer, diabetes, and high cholesterol than Caucasian women, who were primarily worried about osteoporosis and cancer. According to the American Cancer Society (2003), when compared to other racial and ethnic groups, African American women are more likely to die of breast cancer, partly due to failure of early detection of the disease. After acknowledging these concerns about prevalence and incidence, how can African American women impact their health?

The matter of appropriate and available health care including options of alternative or nontraditional care are associated with the issue of informed consent. By actively engaging in the informed consent process, our health and well-being are less likely to be compromised by us due to lack of information, unfamiliarity with medical conditions, feelings of intimidation, and a host of other excuses. Therefore, we can take advantage of those discipline specific standards of protection and safeguards by asking appropriate questions about such issues as contraindications of medication, complications of surgery, side effects of drugs, potential risks and harms of medical procedures or alternative forms of care. Unfortunately, we generally make decisions based on limited information, out of ignorance or due to our perceived sense of intimidation by health care practitioners. Neither ignorance nor naiveté are acceptable excuses when it comes to the application of informed consent and health.

This chapter is not a comprehensive review of the informed consent topic. It is written as an overview to expose the reader to informed decision making and the informed consent process as it applies to personal health and health care. The purpose of this chapter is to empower African American women about the need for decisions to be based on informed consent rather than out of fear, emotions, intimidation or lack of knowledge. The issue of health provides the context for our discussion. However, the process of informed consent as discussed in this chapter has application to a multitude of life situations beyond health and health care, wherever an informed decision is warranted (i.e., special education of children, therapeutic intervention, counseling, placement for an aged parent, etc.). Informed decision making should be the norm and not the exception for informed consent. Remember, informed consent is a process and not just a signoff recorded on paper. Therefore, this chapter addresses the requisites of informed consent, namely, information, understanding of information, communication, autonomy, and trust.

INFORMATION

One might argue that if you have no prior experience or lack familiarity with an illness or disease, how can you possibly give informed consent or make informed decisions about health matters? Being aware of information, having access to information, and understanding the information are elements central to the informed consent process. Information translates into knowledge. In a study by Donovan and Tucker (2000) on knowledge of breast cancer and genetic risk for breast cancer, they found a significant difference in knowledge between African American women and Caucasian women. In comparison, African American women knew significantly less about this disease and their risks for the disease. Without information, African American women will be less likely to make informed decisions about their health or give fully informed consent for treatment.

The importance of the need to have information before consenting is further emphasized by Finger (2002), who describes informed consent as a "more formal, legal process in which the individual is first fully informed and then gives consent, usually in writing" (p. 1). Although he differentiates between informed consent and informed choice, Finger is very clear about the interrelationship between the two concepts and processes. According to Finger (2002), informed choice refers to "ensuring that each client has the information about methods and services—including their risks and benefits that enables clients to make a fully informed decision about whether to obtain or decline treatment or services" (p. 1).

A review by Allen (2000) of traditional models of decision making indicates that people may have a distorted picture of reality due to inadequate information. In such cases, decisions are made under less than optimal circumstances and may be problematic. Therefore, discrepancies in interpretation are likely to exist due to existing knowledge, limited knowledge, or inaccurate information.

When confronted with health issues and crises, we typically defer judgment and rely on the health care provider to either recommend appropriate care or provide us with the necessary information for making complex decisions.

Sometimes, we yield or relinquish responsibility for our welfare by providing blind consent to medical professionals and fail to explore other options. Our dependence on health care providers as the sole source of information is not sufficient for making informed decisions for informed consent. It is critical that other sources of information are identified and considered. Alternative sources may include family and kinship networks, reference groups, social supports, consultation with other specialists, reliable and valid Internet resources, and others.

In everyday life, the active engagement of the safeguards and protections for informed consent, as discussed above, is not without question. Uskul et al. (2003) studied how women made decisions to undergo hysterectomy. They found that women acquired majority of their information about the presentation of their condition and potential treatments through deliberate discussions with other women and that thorough conversations about the pros and cons of alternative treatments did not originate with their physicians. Only the women who became self-informed and sought information on their own engaged in dialog with their gynecologist about alternatives to hysterectomy.

UNDERSTANDING INFORMATION

It should be noted that information alone does not guarantee informed consent. The possession of information does not mean comprehension of the information. According to Fuller et al. (2002), capacity to consent is also need for informed consent, "an individual must be able to understand and retain information regarding treatment" (p. 543). This understanding also extends to benefits and consequences of treatment.

Information should be conveyed in a context that is respectful of cultural, linguistic, and familial orientations of the patient. The literature on information processing addresses the issue of assimilating new information, particularly in relatively brief periods of time. In general, we are less likely to process significant amounts of information during those critical periods when informed consent is required. Therefore, information concerning critical health and serious medical care need to be presented in an understandable manner that is clear, concise, and relevant to the matter.

Our understanding of information necessary for informed decisions about health and related health issues is predicated on one's ability to process the information received and evaluate that information. Evaluating the information for informed consent in a health context must encompass implications of services, treatment, and procedures, as well as, risks and benefits. Therefore, information is clearly necessary but not sufficient for ensuring informed decisions or fully informed consent.

In matters of preventive health care, particularly cancer screening, it should not be assumed that women would automatically comply based on the promotion of screening benefits. Comprehensive information about the benefits and potential harms of screening, along with an understanding of illness and disease are essential for informed consent. The limitations of screening relative to benefits, deleterious effects, and prevention of illness need to be fully understood in order for women to make informed choices (Jepson et al., 2005; Thornton et al., 2003).

The patient bears the responsibility for becoming educated, enlightened, and "informed" about health and health care. Although some may perceive this responsibility as being mutual with the physician, ultimately, it is the responsibility of the patient or consumer to seek the necessary information and to develop an adequate level of understanding sufficient for making an informed decision. The search for information external to the health provider in no way negates the role of the practitioner or diminishes the patient-physician relationship.

COMMUNICATION

Informed consent is a process that begs for opportunities for conversations between a woman and her health care provider. Not simply one conversation but as many discussions as necessary for the establishment of a clear understanding about health issues. Communication is a collaborative effort between a woman and her physician in order for both parties to develop an understanding of each other, awareness of patient concerns, along with issues that impact on the physiological, psychological, social, and environmental well-being of the woman. For example, in their study on breast cancer and genetic risk, Donovan and Tucker (2000) noted that African American women's psychological, social, and economic concerns were different from Caucasian women. Therefore, communication between African American women and their health practitioner must be individualized and culturally sensitive to the needs of the specific patient.

For fully informed consent to exist, communication between African American women and their physicians must go beyond the superficial "doctor knows best" relationship. Although social convention may dictate accepting what the physician tells you, history demands that women assert themselves and assume a different type of role with health care practitioners. For example, if the woman has the interest and intellect to read medical literature concerning the health issue in question, the physician should provide the woman with those resources for review and contemplation. Based on this type of exchange of information, invited followup discussions would be most appropriate and beneficial for the process of informed consent. An informed consent model by Widdershoven and Verheggen (1999) focuses on the role of communication between patient and physician and on mutual decision making. Their model promotes the active engagement of patients in the decision making process concerning medical matters.

Communication between a patient and practitioner is a two-way process. Communication that is characterized by the sharing of information in a comprehensible manner and clarification of terminology and other germane information are essential to the informed consent process. The communication needs to be an intentional, didactic, ongoing process designed to garner support on both sides, while building a sense of trust, openness, and mutual respect.

TRUST

There is a growing body of literature on the lack of participation of African American women in medical research and clinical trials, and the underlying concerns regarding trust (Freimuth et al., 2001; Freedman, 1998; Gamble, 1997; Harris et al., 1996). For example, African American women in the Freedman (1998) study "feared that a white doctor might not have knowledge and understanding of the health problems faced by black people from a biological and a life situation perspective, and might not know what to look for in a black patient" (p. 944).

Unlike the African American women in the Freedman (1998) study, many women fail to voice their similar concerns about health care practices and relationships with health providers. Perhaps informed consent should be conceptualized as an empowering opportunity for African American women to take responsibility for their own health and welfare by actively participating in the management of their health; engaging in relevant discussions about health; being persistent in the quest to develop a more in-depth understanding; making informed decisions about services, treatments, and procedures; raising issues and questions about health; and exploring alternatives of care as needed. In reality, informed decisions and informed consent raise the level of accountability and responsibility for both the patient and the practitioner, and can result in a trusting relationship.

Despite the fact that we entrust physicians and other health providers with our care, women should not adopt a passive role. Women need to be deliberate and intentional in their choice of physicians. It is important for African American women to review references and consult social networks when searching for and selecting new health care professionals. Women also need to revive relationships with existing practitioners, in light of their active engagement of informed decision making. Health care practitioners for African American women need to be sensitive to the cultural and spiritual orientations of the patient for the promotion of trust and mutual respect.

Given that informed consent is not just a legal activity designed to protect the health care provider, it is a process that promotes accountability of care and patient-provider communication. Informed consent has the potential to engender a trusting relationship between a woman and her health professional. When a patient and physician assume shared accountability and responsibility for the health and welfare of the patient, a partnership develops, whether formal or informal in nature. However, there is a tremendous need for some level of rapport to be developed in order to foster that partnership. Rapport is crucial to the communication process and establishes the foundation for the partnership, whether or not persons are similar in cultural and ethnic background.

Partnerships between women and their health care providers are cultivated over time and enhance the communication process. However, rapport building is a dynamic process that should occur throughout the relationship. Essential to the partnership is mutual respect for one another and trust, along with rejection of the myth that the doctor knows best. As partners with mutual interests in the health and well-being of the patient, the health care system can be appreciative of a woman's personal knowledge about her health and body.

NATURE OF CONSENT

A discussion on informed consent is not complete without attention being paid to the nature of consent. Although consent is perceived by most people to be voluntary in nature, some might suggest that consent relative to health care may be somewhat coerced. However, as defined by the ethical practices, standards, and guidelines of professional associations, informed consent is voluntary. Voluntariness, also referred to as autonomy, is a requirement for informed consent (Strauss et al., 2001).

The provision of relevant information to the patient does not guarantee the voluntariness of consent. Women may give consent to their health care practitioners, but they may not fully understand the scope of the implications or comprehend the nature of their consent (Finger, 2002). Research on this topic also indicates that some patients feel they have no other choice and therefore, simply go along to prevent losing services or medical care. For example, Joubert, Steinberg, van der Ryst, and Chikobvu (2003) examined the voluntariness of informed consent of women in a Bloemfontein vitamin A trial. They found that 3.3 percent of the women reported feeling coerced to participate, 24.2 percent believed they could withdraw from the study, and 92.3 percent perceived that withdrawal would eliminate their quality medical care.

Language and culture may impede the process of informed consent. Different cultural beliefs and customs associated health practices, treatment, or services may be viewed as being in conflict with traditional health care. Differing values and beliefs of both the patient and practitioner may be misinterpreted, perceived as competitive or even considered distrustful of the health care system.

Although patients may solicit recommendations from their physicians, the final decision to accept or refuse service or treatment, rests with the woman. Refusal to consent to unclear or unfamiliar health services or treatment may be perceived by some as a lack of compliance on the part of the patient. However, based on informed consent, the patient may simply be exercising her right for clarification and further scrutiny before making a serious decision.

Moreover, the timing of the presentation of information may also interfere with the informed consent process. In the midst of a health crisis, a woman may feel overwhelmed by receipt of too much information in conjunction with the demand for written consent. The perceived or real pressure from the health care system may further exacerbate the problem of trust and respect between the woman and the health care provider.

RECOMMENDATIONS

African American women need to pause and determine how they actually make decisions about their personal health and health care. Through a reflective process, women can discern whether they actively participate in the decision-making process or simply acquiesce to recommendations from their primary care physician or other health care providers.

Decisions regarding health matters need to be based on informed consent and not speculation, fear, pressure or ignorance. Women need to render consent on the basis of accurate, valid, and complete information. Therefore, it is important to determine if you engage in the informed consent process with your physician or other health care providers. This can be assessed by objectively examining the relationship and evaluating comfort levels, receptivity to questions, and nature of explanations.

Consider the following questions as you reflect on whether you practice informed consent when making health care decisions:

Are you fully informed about your health status?

Are you cognizant of the implications of treatment for your condition?

What alternative treatments exist for your medical problem?

Are they relevant for your particular case?

What are the common and atypical side effects of your medication?

What information did your physician provide about your illness?

What other sources of information are you aware of?

Where did you go for a second opinion about a recent diagnosis?

Who else in your family has this medical condition?

These questions are central to a discussion between a patient and her physician in order for the patient to make informed health decisions necessary for informed consent.

Informed consent is a process, not just access to information. Given that information alone is not sufficient for informed consent, the following actions have been identified to encourage women to consciously engage in the informed consent process, as part of their decision making for health matters:

- Invest in yourself by making your health a priority.
- Take responsibility for your health by engaging in healthy lifestyles and health-enhancing behaviors.
- Identify and select primary care physicians with care and discernment, ensuring they are appreciative of your cultural and spiritual orientations.
- Develop a partnership with your primary care physician that is built on trust, mutual respect, and communication.
- Initiate conversations with health care providers about your health status and health care.
- Empower yourself with information and knowledge.
- Be diligent in your search for information and use reliable, valid resources, including electronic information systems.
- Develop a network of people you trust to serve as personal health care advocates and consultants.

- Make informed decisions by asking questions about benefits and harms, contra-indications, alternative services and treatments, and so forth.

SUMMARY

African American women have responsibility for making significant decisions about their lives and the lives of their loved ones. Among these numerous decisions are those concerning their personal health and health related matters. How and when these decisions are made and under what conditions are the real questions needing answers.

As African American women suffer from chronic and life-threatening illness and disease, attention needs to be focused on how decisions are made about services and treatment. The process of informed consent can serve as a tool for ensuring that health decisions are deliberate, thoughtful, and in the best interest of the woman. Although derived from concern for protecting human participants in research, the process of informed consent has application to health care. Parallel safeguards and guidelines for informed consent exist in the health care industry to protect patients requiring procedures, services or treatment. Fully informed consent mandates that all necessary information is available to the patient, including benefits and potential harms, implications of treatment, alternative procedures, services, and treatments in order to render an informed decision. However, discussions about informed consent within the everyday context of patient-physician relationships may not be as commonplace as compared to humans consenting to participate in research.

Informed consent is not a onetime event but an ongoing process between a woman and her health care professional. Requisites of informed consent include information, understanding of information, communication, trust, and personal autonomy. Informed consent needs to be grounded in information, voluntary in nature, and based on the patient's ability to make intelligent and informed decisions.

The process of informed consent challenges African American women to be knowledgeable about their bodies and health status, persistent in their search for information, and accountable and responsible for maintaining healthy lifestyles and establishing partnerships with health care professionals. In other words, African American women need to transform their concern about health and potential disease into actions reflective of health-enhancing behaviors rather than health-compromising behaviors. Making deliberate choices about lifestyles, seeking pertinent information, searching for appropriate resources, and engaging in daily health practices that promote well-being are all actions indicative of informed decisions.

True informed consent really means that you fully understand what you are consenting to, why you are granting consent, and the implications of consent for your life. *So, when was the last time you gave informed consent about a health matter?* The answer to this question is not the end of this chapter, but only the beginning!

REFERENCES

Allen, R. F. January/February 2000. "Civic Education and the Decision-making Process." *The Social Studies,* 91(1):5.

American Cancer Society. 2003. *Cancer Statistics, 2003.* New York: Lippincott Williams & Wilkins.

American College of Obstetricians and Gynecologists. 1989. *Informed Consent.* Washington, DC: The College and The Assistant, ACOG, Department of Professional Liability.

American Medical Association. 1997. *Code of Medical Ethics.* Chicago: American Medical Association.

American Psychological Association. 2002. *Ethical Principles of Psychologists and Code of Conduct.* Accessed June 16, 2005, from http://www.apa.org/ethics/code2002.html.

Annas, G. I. 1998. *Some Choice: Law, Medicine, and the Market.* New York: Oxford University Press.

Donovan, K. A., and D. C. Tucker. February 2000. "Knowledge about Genetic Risk for Breast cancer and Perceptions of Genetic Testing in a Sociodemographically Diverse Sample." *Journal of Behavioral Medicine,* 23(1):15–36.

Finger, W. R. 2002. "Choices Must Be Informed, Voluntary." *Network,* 21, no. 2, Accessed March 18, 2005, from http://thi.org/en/RH/Pubs/Network/v21_2/NW21-2informconst.htm.

Finkelstein, E. A., O. A. Khavjou, L. R. Mobley, D. M. Haney, and J. C. Will. June 2004. "Racial/ethnic Disparities in Coronary Heart Disease Risk Factors Among WISEWOMAN Enrollees." *Journal of Women's Health,* 13(5):503–518.

Freedman, T. G. October 1998. "Why Don't They Come to Pike Street and Ask Us?: Black American Women's Health Concerns." *Social Science and Medicine,* 47 (7):941–947.

Freimuth, V. S., S. Quinn, S. B. Thomas, G. Cole, E. Zook, and T. Duncan. March 2001. "African American's Views on Research and the Tuskegee Syphilis Study." *Social Science and Medicine,* 52(5):797–808.

Fuller, R., N. Dudley, and J. Blacktop. September 2002. "How Informed Is Consent?: Understanding of Pictorial and Verbal Probability Information by Medical Inpatients." *Postgraduate Medical Journal,* 78(923):543.

Gamble, V. 1997. "Under the Shadow of Tuskegee: African Americans and Health Care." *American Journal of Public Health,* 87, 1773–1778.

Goldzieher, J. W., L. Moses, E. Averkin, C. Scheel, and B. Taber. 1971. "A Placebo-controlled Double-blind Crossover Investigation of the Side Effects Attributed to Oral Contraceptives." *Fertility and Sterility,* 22(9):609–623.

Harris, Y., P. H. Gorelick, P. Samuels, and I. Bempong. 1996. "Why African Americans May Not Be Participating in Clinical Trials." *Journal of the National Medical Association,* 88, 630–634.

Jepson, R. G., J. Hewison, A.G.H. Thompson, and D. Weller. April 2005. "How Should We Measure Informed Choice? The Case of Cancer Screening." *Journal of Medical Ethics,* 31(4):192–196. Accessed June 3, 2005, from http://web22.epnet.com/citation.asp?tb=1&_ug=sid+54B6D68F%2DA85F%2D42A5%2DB.

Joubert, G., H. Steinberg, E. van der Ryst, and P. Chikobvu. April 2003. "Consent for Participation in the Bloemfontein Vitamin A Trial: How Informed and Voluntary?" *American Journal of Public Health,* 93(4):582–584.

National Commission for the Protection of Human Subjects of Biomedical and Behavioral Research. 1979. *The Belmont Report: Ethical Principles and Guidelines for the Protection of Human subjects of Research.* Washington, DC: Author. Accessed June 5, 2005, from http://ohsr.od.nih.gov/mpa/belmont.php3.

Nelson-Marten, P., and B. A. Rich. 1999. "A Historical Perspective of Informed Consent in Clinical Practice and Research." *Seminars in Oncology Nursing*, 15(2):81–88.

Pikler, V., and C. Winterowd. November 2003. "Racial and Body Image Differences in Coping for Women Diagnosed with Breast Cancer." *Health Psychology*, 22(6): 632–637.

Stover, J. C., A. H. Skelly, D. Holditch-Davis, and P. F. Dunn. May 2001. "Perceptions of Health and Their Relationship to Symptoms in African American Women with Type 2 Diabetes." *Applied Nursing Research*, 14(2):72–80.

Strauss, R., S. Sengupta, S. Quinn, J. Goeppinger, C. Spaulding, S. Kegeles, and G. Millett. December 2001. "The Role of Community Advisory Boards: Involving Communities in the Informed Consent Process." *American Journal of Public Health*, 91(12):1938–1943.

Thornton, H., A. Edwards, and M. Baum. July 2003. "Women Need Better Information about Routine Mammography." *British Medical Journal*, 327(7406):101–103. Accessed June 3, 2005, from http://web22.epnet.com/citation.asp?tb=1&_ug=sid+54B6D68F%2DA85F%2DA.

U.S. Department of Health and Human Services. 1991. *Protection of Human Subjects*. 45 CFR 46, Rockville, MD: Author. Accessed May 26, 2005, from http://www.hrsa.gov/quality/hsrtraining.htm.

Uskul, A. K., F. Ahmad, N. A. Leyland, and D. E. Stewart. 2003. "Women's Hysterectomy Experiences and Decision-making." *Women and Health*, 38(1):53.

Widdershoven, G., and F. Verheggen. July–August 1999. "Improving Informed Consent by Implementing Shared Decisionmaking in Health Care." *A Review of Human Subjects Research*, 21(4):1–4.

Wilcox, S., B. E. Ainsworth, M. J. LaMonte, and K. D. DuBose. November 2002. "Worry Regarding Major Diseases among Older African American, Native American, and Caucasian Women." *Women and Health*, 36(3):83.

12

Women in the Shadows: Seeking Health, Seeking Self

VIRGINIA A. BATCHELOR

If you ask any African American woman about her personal experiences, she will tell you, "Life is a struggle. I have to fight everybody, everywhere, for everything." Ask her what she yearns for and she will tell you, "Love, honor, and respect." Growing up in the United States as an African American girl is particularly difficult. As a woman, by dominant cultural standards, she will be perceived and depicted as both immoral and yet a towering pillar of strength (Ladner, 1995). This chapter arises out of a particular context of being perceived as the "other" among both familiar and unfamiliar faces. Catholic school experiences have had a major impact upon Black womanhood. These experiences were both challenging and at times, painful at best, for me, and the women that I encountered on my journey in the shadows. The shadow is symbolic of prejudice. Prejudice as explained by W.E.B. Du Bois (1994) is a series of antithetical relationships that deems, for example, one culture and/or ethnicity superior and the other inferior. Therefore, in the face of prejudice, inevitably, self-doubt and self-disparagement sets in to devalue prior knowledge, beliefs, and values. Further, Du Bois views prejudice as a natural defense of the prevailing culture. To this end, the prevailing culture strives to maintain its position of power as the standard for all cultures, and thus regards other cultures as "barbaric." Consequently, these women felt they had to rely upon their cultural strengths to construct survival strategies in order to affirm themselves in two separate environments. In the community, the women had to prove they had not abandoned their culture; in their Catholic schooling experience, they had to defend their culture legitimate and worthy alongside dominant cultural values. As African American women, the constant challenge of proving the validity of their personhood among the familiar and unfamiliar faces is the central theme of this work.

For many African American women, while they struggle to lead their families and be the strength of their communities, much of their personal "selves" are left neglected. However, there comes a time to contemplate one's personal self, to reckon with one's past, and come to terms with one's personal truth outside of societal views. I therefore ventured into the shadows to tune into the multiple voices and expressions of survival to make sense of the self as illuminated through the experiences of African American women.

BACKGROUND

This chapter examines the racial perceptions experienced by nineteen African American women in the Catholic secondary education system. The narrations were collected over a period of twenty-four months. These "womanist" experiences were reproduced informally across American kitchens, living rooms, and any space or location where two or more Black women gathered together to seek support.

Gleaned from the women's point of view is the socialization process of how Eurocentric cultural constructs of race, gender, class, and religion impact African cultural forms among African American girls in, for instance, Catholic schools. In other words, it examines the effects of what is referred to as "culture shock" within these systems of domination. Also included is how gender ideology within the context of Catholicism reinforced female inferiority. This socialization process reaches an even more devastating level for African American women as a result of multiple systems of dominance (e.g., cultural hegemony, plus race, class, and gender oppression) that contribute to a social identity that imposes negative self-concepts on them.

The underrepresentation of African American women in major American social institutions and the historic legacy of oppression in the United States combine to create a sense of personal devaluation and loss of self-esteem. Although this chapter centers on African American women within the context of Catholicism, overall, these negative experiences can be generalizable to the Black female experience in American society. For the purpose of this chapter, I will examine some of their stressors and identify coping strategies they used to survive these negative experiences.

To best explain the social, spiritual, historical, and cultural context of African American women's experiences, I utilized African and woman-centered theories. These theories illuminates the importance of sisterhood and the nurturing spirit of motherhood that Black women extend to one another as a means of spiritual and emotional support. Additionally, the experiences of these women will serve to raise consciousness and bring awareness that some individuals or groups do not experience equal status or equity in school, the workplace, or in the greater society. Acknowledgment of this pain increases awareness. Awareness, the impetus for understanding other lived realities will hopefully touch the hearts and minds of women who occupy both spaces of power and subordination and who perpetuate such inequalities (i.e., women oppressing other women).

A JOURNEY INTO THE SHADOW

African American women have served to be the backdrop of society. They occupy spaces in the shadows only to be brought to the forefront to exemplify or illustrate "what is deviant." The notion of being in the shadows speaks to the heart of African American women. Therefore, one must journey into the shadows and tune into the multiple voices there. Sometimes, it is through others that one comes to a deeper understanding of oneself.

African American women oftentimes feel that they are deemed insignificant; that is in the "shadow." How past experiences of being the "other" within their community as well as within their Catholic high schools was a conversation long overdue. These women felt it was important to make sense of the past as a means of reconciling the present. To this end, it is necessary to provide a context for understanding the culture and the community from where these voices were found.

THERE'S NO PLACE LIKE HOME: HOME IS WHERE THE HEART IS

The community (home) is where the heart is. Therefore, it is hurtful to experience alienation and isolation within one's community. The community is where its people construct meaning of their lives based upon beliefs and values. It is within the community that the day-to-day experiences shape the social identity (i.e., Black identity and Black consciousness) of Black families, children and men and women.

Some of the members of the African American community perceived all or most African Americans who were Catholic or attended Catholic schools as wealthy and elitist. Although these women described themselves as working class, they experienced resentment because they were perceived to have undeserved wealth. Therefore, anything having to do with Catholicism, particularly Catholic schooling created stress. For example, Samaria described a childhood incident as bordering on assault because she attended a Catholic school.

I was an "only" child and it appeared to a lot of people that I had certain privileges that others did not have. It was pretty exaggerated 'cause it also felt that way in the Catholic school as well. There were a couple young men on the street that took to calling me "Catlic" and, actually, sought to ambush me a couple of times to toss me [back and forth] with the "Catlic" girl, "Catlic" School, "Catlic" school. . . . It was almost bordering on assault, you know. They just never got to that point, but they were one step away from actually assaulting me over this Catholic school and calling me "Catlic." . . . The poor little rich girl.

Although, according to Samaria, the teasing and taunting did not become physically abusive to the extent of sustaining injury; nonetheless, it was a frightening experience that left her feeling emotionally and physically unsafe among familiar faces (people in the community). Imani expressed similar experiences.

I had a problem because I lived in a neighborhood where the other Black children did not go to Catholic school. So I had to fight where I was, and fight where I went to school.

P. H. Collins (1991) examined the role of the outsider within. Within this framework, these Black women who attended predominately white institutions were outsiders by virtue of their blackness or the biological representations of race. In other words, they were not denied access to these schools, however they were denied privileges afforded to whites within these schools. With respect to their position in the community, they were insider/outsider within. That is, within the community, they were insiders because they shared a culture and history, as well as they were Black girls. However, as Black girls attending predominately white institutions, they lost full group membership among the members within their community thus deeming them "outsiders within." As a result, the position as outcast in both worlds substantiated their subordination, thus creating stress.

When the Shadow Swept across Me

Ironically, high school experiences mirrored the professional lives of these women. They expressed that high school was very much an adult experience. In other words, they felt that children should not be exposed to, for example, racist behavior within a religious-based institution. As Deka put it: "One of five African Americans in an all-white school was definitely an experience." Additionally, being outnumbered within the workplace presented similar stressors. As students in school, they felt singled out for reprimands and overlooked for praises. As women in the workplace, they noted they were welcome to share in the struggle to improve employee benefits; but overlooked for promotions and raises.

Tyler (one of the many voices in the shadows) expressed that as a member of an underrepresented group within a religious-based school, she felt a racist element. Consequently, it was a major focus in and upon the lives of the African American students. According to Tyler, it was not until high school that she was affected on a personal level by attitudes of indifference based upon race. As a Black Catholic, it was an interesting lesson because (Catholic or non-Catholic), a spirit of acceptance between the African American students and the nuns was missing. The following excerpts illustrate diversity within the Catholic high schools. Tyler exclaimed:

In our class, there were five! Five Black people in the class! When there's only five of you, what difference does it make? We're not going to take over the school. What are you so afraid of? I felt like in many instances like the little token "Negroes." Well you know, we do have, so they would say at their meetings.... We have five Negro girls and they're very lovely you know.

According to Imani: "You could count how many Blacks were in the school on one hand." More often than not, one can count the number of African Americans in "certain" schools as well, in positions of power within the workplace. For the most part, Black women express that attitudes have not changed in terms of being fearful of two or more African Americans socializing. As Tyler put it, "What are they so afraid of?" However, painful, the Catholic schooling experience was considered basic training for life.

Stereotypical views of African American women as deviants create stress. Childhood experiences impact adult self-concepts positively or negatively. As adults, these women are haunted still, by childhood misperceptions of having undeserved wealth and a superiority complex (among familiar faces). The workplace is the school environment minus the perceived spiritual element.

Deka expressed that her Catholic school experience prepared her in terms of coping in situations where she is the only African American or only woman. Although a lack of diversity is still prevalent in many situations, especially the workplace, these women felt far more prepared to meet the demands of their professional lives and advance professionally because they had been exposed to people from different cultural backgrounds.

Within the walls of the Catholic schools, academic success was a priority. The same holds true in the workplace. Top performance is a major focus and the feeling of having to be "better than" by virtue of one's skin tone is a burden. Their past experiences revealed that friendships were difficult to maintain within the community; and friendships in school were difficult to establish due to the environment, which perpetuated stereotypical views of African Americans. Consequently, Black women find they have to negotiate their place within various spaces in society; and at times in sites where there is acceptance and resistance.

LESSONS LEARNED AS GIRLS: WHY [DO] YOU TREAT ME SO BAD?

Initial experiences, like, the first day of school or the first day on a new job determines how one feels about the situation at hand and themselves. According to Cooley (1902), individuals interpret the reactions of others toward them and therefore judge themselves according to how they perceive others see and judge them. If for instance, the individual experiences acceptance, a positive self-concept is likely to develop. Conversely, rejection diminishes positive self-concepts.

African American women wonder why they are most often targeted for abuse. As girls and as women, the question that remains unanswered is: Why [do] you treat me so bad? After taking a deep breath as if to inhale memories from her past, Deka experienced and believed African American students were not welcome in the Catholic school she attended. The tradition of the school was totally European. The perception was that anything outside of that was unacceptable and inferior.

Racial or ethnic cliques arise out of cultural differences due to the lack of understanding. However, most striking was what Samaria experienced and also stated: "They did something to us. I don't know what it was. I can't explain it but they did something to us." To make sense of what "they" did or did not do, it is important to examine the impact of the doctrine and practices of the Catholic Church on the Catholic sisterhood. Within this tradition lies a deeper understanding of the nuns' role in how they shaped the cultural identity and self-concepts of African American girls in the Catholic schools; and the subsequent impact of the experience of it upon their lives.

SHAPING THE SISTERHOOD: THE DOCTRINE AND PRACTICES OF THE CATHOLIC CHURCH

The nuns as the primary and most important authority figures in Catholic schools advanced a Catholic culture that deemed women inferior over men. With respect to convent training, women of the religious tradition (nuns) took three vows: poverty, obedience, and chastity (Coburn & Smith, 1999). Although these women used their vows to justify their public endeavors and positions, otherwise held by men to minister to the members in the community, a religious life required that women be silent. That is, convent training promoted a life of discipline and character to withstand "potentially primitive conditions, loneliness, isolation, at times grinding poverty and emotional disappointment" (Coburn & Smith, 1999, p. 75). This religious ideology shaped American Catholic culture and therefore shaped the culture of the Catholic schools.

And the socialization process that took place in the Catholic high schools perpetuated and further prepared these girls to endure emotional disappointment and loneliness as women. Olufemi described her childhood memories as having few friendships. For the most part, her sister was, and is still, her best friend. She explained: "We went to school. We had no friends. It was kind of lonely. We were two lonely children, but we didn't realize it."

The day-to-day stresses of isolation and alienation made growing up difficult. Surviving these experiences as girls was painful, at best and consequently, these stresses rolled over into other relationships as women (e.g., personal, spiritual, and professional lives). Presently, small circles of friends, mostly from similar childhood experiences make up the world of these women.

EXAMINING CULTURAL STANDARDS: IN SEARCH OF "SELF"

In an interesting intersection of systematic oppression within a religious-based school, African American girls were cast as social deviants in relation to the student body. As Hazika put it, "We were marked." This perceived deviance made them vulnerable to emotional, psychological, and spiritual attack. Evaluation under the influence of the nuns, such as one's conduct values, and self-perceptions in terms of a religious-based morality, suggested character annihilation.

Comparisons between past experiences as girls to present experiences as women were consistent. For instance, in the Catholic high school environment, the women felt they were perceived in relation to Euro-American girls as "transgressors," as opposed to "virtuous" women (Riggs, 1993). Some of the women compared the Catholic high school to the workplace in that they were referred to as "trouble-makers" in both sites.

An emphasis upon ranking and categorizations creates antithetical relationships (i.e., privileging versus demoralizing). Consequently, African American girls felt devalued and disrespected by the nuns. Stereotypes that perpetuated cultural clashes further deem African American women a marginalized group both as the "other" or immoral. As Journey explained, the perceptions of African American girls were obviously different from the white girls. She states: "You know . . . that Blacks aren't into anything. You know . . . we were this and we were that. We were just into sex." Samaria also thought the nuns perceived African Americans as immoral and as underachievers. The ways in which nuns related to her, case in point, gestures, tone of voice and insensitive comments such as "you people" made their distance clear.

Noted from girlhood experiences, the women expressed that the environment of the Catholic high schools did not promote self-pride nor pride in one's heritage. As Father Lawrence E. Lucas (a Black Catholic priest) sums it up:

From my earliest experiences in the Catholic Church, the virtues drummed into me in school, convert classes, etc., were nonviolence, obedience, humility, love, patience, forgiveness of enemies, long-suffering and hope in a future reward, but not in this life. Rarely did I hear about the other virtues of self-esteem, pride, gratitude to God for what we are (rather than gratitude for the ability to become, if not white, then gray or colored), legitimate self-defense, just anger, liberty and freedom, the right to share in Our Father's earthly goods in this life. (1992, pp. 86–87)

All in all, the Catholic school was an institution that did not provide a culturally affirming environment. Moreover, when there is a dominance of one culture, there is a tendency to exclude people in the minority from sharing in the advantages afforded to the majority culture (Hacker, 1992).

In general, messages of inferiority are found throughout women's culture. For African American women, societal standards are filled with astonishing amounts of distortions that create and advance classist, racialized, and genderized ideologies. Amina believed that the attitudes of the nuns expressed a sense of superiority.

They thought that we were inferior. Well, I thought they thought we were inferior . . . that we couldn't accomplish things. It made you feel as though you were inferior. And to accept, someone, somebody [telling us] that they can expect less an accomplishment because of who we are . . . whatever. . . . But I never let that stop me from doing what I had to do.

In addition, the nuns as women negotiated their societal roles (dominant and subordinate) within the gendered power dynamics of religious traditions (Coburn & Smith, 1999) emerging as fragmented beings; inferior because they were women and superior because they were white. In other words, the nuns were also manipulated by societal myths to become what Freire (1993) refers to as "fundamental instruments for the preservation of domination" (p. 129).

Domination is oppressive. Domination within the context of religion is emotionally wounding. The nuns were oppressed by their gender and class and the girls were oppressed by their gender, class, and race. As Freire informs us, it is necessary to examine the roles of the oppressed and the oppressor. Not only does the oppressor inauthenticate the oppressed accordingly the oppressed becomes more like the oppressor. Neither role produces a healthy sense of self. Oppression breeds a spirit of aggression that I refer to as hagarenism.

Hagarenism, an outgrowth of oppression is sketched in the biblical text of Genesis 16:1–16. Two women, Hagar and Sarah, both of whom are oppressed by their gender, although Sarah is privileged by her class, reveal a catastrophic form of oppression at the hands of a woman with a false sense of power over her "sister." Hagarenism illustrate relationships whereby an individual or group seeks to have their needs met to gain or maintain control through the exploitation of oppressed individuals. This type of aggression is verbal and emotionally violent and therefore attacks the spirit of an individual. In order to heal Hagar, it is of central importance to know and love one's true self.

AFRICAN AMERICAN WOMEN: SEEKING HEALTH THROUGH SEEKING SELF

The shared experiences of these women served to be a means of changing the perceptions of their own realities. Their experiences were presented to me within a cultural context that embodied their vision of who they were as girls and who they are as women. By examining their past, they created a path to their true sense of self. Additionally, examination of the past diminished self-blaming and thus provided a deeper understanding of the experiences that took place. Their collective voices served to rewrite our stories and leave behind a model that resuscitated a dormant self that was alive and worthy of a space within the larger community of women.

One thing for certain is that African American women are resilient. They love hard and unconditionally. They have heart and soul that is so welcoming that other oppressed groups seek them out for refuge. They are temples, and deserving to be covered by the power and protection of God. They use their strength to be a fashionable comforter that they appropriate for public and private use. They are not afraid to reveal her vulnerability.

African American women are gifted interpreters of their environment. They are experts in reinventing themselves for survival sake. As C. F. Collins (2003) explains, African American women wear many hats—each having the potential to create stress.

First, with respect to minority status within various institutional structures, African American women project a self that ensures acceptance among other African Americans as well as among members of the dominant culture. According to Gibson (1988), by assuming the appropriate behavior according to the circumstances at the time, African American women demonstrate a proficiency in the norms and behaviors of both cultures.

Central to African American women's survival are friendships. Genuine sisterhood that fosters self-acceptance and renders emotional support served to relieve stress.

Naming is an important element of African woman-centered theories in that it is empowering. Given that naming is the voice of empowerment, participation is encouraged in, for example, church activities, cultural clubs, and community organizations. By engaging in intellectual exchanges, African American women find spaces in which to discuss issues impacting the lived realities of African Americans as well as utilize these discussions to deconstruct negative images and reconstruct positive self-definitions. By redefining our sense of self within our vision, we transcend the limitations that systems of domination such as race, gender, and class impose upon marginalized people (Collins, 1991; Batchelor, 2001).

Finally, most important to African American women's survival has been, and is still, their sense of spirituality. Letting go and letting God free us of the stressors and frustrations from the past weeks by engaging in a "Holy Ghost" dance of shouting and singing fuels the spirit to make it through another day, week, month, or year. Within our "purist" sense of spirituality, African American women become truly moral, and therefore possess a sense of being that is acceptable and deserving of God's love. In other words, from the soul's remembrance of what it means to be in touch with one's authentic self, the "self" in its purest state is in balance with God. Given that, social and self-affirming constructs emerge, and all else becomes less important.

REFERENCES

Batchelor, V. A. 2001. *Those Catholic School Girls*. UMI Dissertation Services. Ann Arbor, MI: Bell & Howell Information and Learning Company.

Coburn, C. K., and M. Smith. 1999. *Spirited Lives: How Nuns Shaped Catholic Culture American Life, 1836–1920*. Chapel Hill, NC: University of North Carolina Press.

Collins, C. F. 2003. *Sources of Stress and Relief for African-American Women*. Westport, CT: Praeger.

Collins, P. H. 1991. *Black Feminist Thought: Knowledge, Consciousness, and the Politics of Empowerment*. New York: Routledge.

Cooley, C. H. 1902. *Human Nature and the Social Order*. New York: Scribner's.

Du Bois, W.E.B. 1994. *The Souls of Black Folk*. Mineola, NY: Dover Publications.

Freire, P. 1993. *Pedagogy of the Oppressed*. New York: Continuum Publishing Company.

Gibson, M. 1988. *Accommodation without Assimilation: Sikh Immigrants In an American High School*. Ithaca, NY: Cornell University Press.

Hacker, A. 1992. *Two nations: Black and White, Separate, Hostile, Unequal*. New York: Ballantine Publishers.

Ladner, J. A. 1995. *Tomorrow's Tomorrow*. Garden City, NY: Doubleday.

Lucas, L. E. 1992. *Black Priest, White Church: Catholics and Racism*. Trenton, NJ: Africa World Press.

Riggs, M. Y. 1993. "A Clarion Call to Awake! Arise! AT!: The Response of the Black
    Women's Club Movement to Institutionalize the Moral Evil." In Emilie Townes
    (Ed.), *A Troubling In My Soul* (pp. 67–77). New York: Maryknoll.
Taylor, H. L., Jr. 1990. *African Americans and the Rise of Buffalo's Post-industrial City,
    1940–present: Volume 1. An Introduction to a Research Report.* Buffalo, NY:
    Buffalo Urban League Inc.

13

Women of Color and the Roots of Coping: A Literary Perspective

IMANI LILLIE B. FRYAR

There are cultural variations in how individuals of different societies handle oppression. Strategies appearing negative to the outside observer may be the appropriate mechanism for the oppressed to repossess or reconnect to their cultural bearings. When African American women were enslaved, various stereotypes were created to define and control their behavior, such as mammy, sapphire, Caldonia, sex-kitten, and so on. However, through literary analysis, I will examine works of African American women from various time periods to illuminate the strategies these women elected as survival techniques, redefining themselves along the way, and how these coping skills are residuals of the African tradition. Some of the works cited are: *Our Nig*, Harriet Wilson; *Incidents in the Life of a Slave Girl*, Linda Brent; *Their Eyes Were Watching God*, Zora Neale Hurston; *Sula*, Toni Morrison; and *Waiting to Exhale*, Terry McMillan. Lena Wright Myers, in her book, *Black Women Do They Cope Better?* (1991, p. 14) states:

Theoretically, it is believed that we learn to think of ourselves as we do, primarily on the basis of how others see us, as shown by their behavior toward us. But not all others count equally. These people who have the most impact upon our self-esteem and attitudes are those we have the most in common with. Our key to coping with racism and sexism . . . was to get an image of ourselves based on how well we do whatever we are doing and how others whose opinion matters to us view our success in whatever we do.

RELIGION AND RITUAL FOR COPING

For Black women, the opinion would be, of course, from other Black women and mother substitutes. In Myers's report, she interviewed 200 Black women from Grand Rapids, Michigan, in 1972; 200 from Jackson, Mississippi, in 1974; and 200 women ten years later from Georgia, Washington, D.C., Illinois, Michigan, Mississippi, and New Jersey. The women interviewed attested to a strong religious connection:

Not only have family ties been a source of strength for Black women, but also the church and the clergy. Since slavery, the church has been a viable institution in the lives of Black people. The views of the Black women in my sample support this contention. The majority of the women felt that the church and religion helped to prepare them for getting ahead in life. Responses as to how the church and religion helped them included: "The Lord would always show me the way to go." "Got to have something to believe in, in order to get ahead, and I believe in spiritual things." (Myers, 1991, p. 28)

While Myers work alludes to W.E.B. Du Bois' (1903, p. 45) theory to living behind the veil, "always seeing ourselves through the eyes of others," Black women in their coping mechanisms have extracted the "others" to be those whom they trust and who know them. So the veil is a positive covering of protection and is important because, as seekers of the truth, they know that those with whom they have spent time and are like them know them best. In the African tradition, the highest motivation for individuals is to know their life purpose and pursue it. People in your community know your purpose also.

In the book *We Have No Word for Sex*, by Malidoma and Sonofu Some (1994), they talk about the ritual that women have of returning once a year with their rites-of-passage initiates to rebond and nurture one another. Sonofu is from the Dagara tribe of Burkina Faso, West Africa. Her name means "keeper of the rituals," and she describes the many gender-specific rituals. Even in the villages, women and men do not sleep together. Women are constantly bonding and learning how to be women from their elders and female relatives; their abilities are reinforced and nurtured by other women. So when they return to the village to carry out these roles, they are fortified and strong.

In the South it was relatively easy to carry out these traditions in agricultural settings, but with industrialization and continued racist and sexist oppression, it became increasingly difficult for Black women to replicate these rituals, and therefore they become isolated. The bond was broken during slavery, and Black women have not completely found their way back yet. However, the many Black female groups such as Delta Sigma Theta, Links, 100 Black Women, Jack & Jill of America, and International Black Women's Congress, to name a few, all serve to help alleviate the pain of isolation, and they are successful. Nevertheless, it is still important to see the connection these groups have to African traditions so that cultural ties will be strong.

In Linda Brent's *Incidents in the Life of a Slave Girl* (1973), Linda's grandmother protected her, most of the time, from the slave master' sexual exploitation. As she ponders her daily battles with Dr. Flint, she reflects:

I longed for someone to confide in. I would have given he world to have laid my head on my grandmother's faithful bosom, and told her all of my troubles. But Dr. Flint swore he would kill me if I was not silent as the grave. Then, although my grandmother was all in all to me, I feared her as well as loved her. . . . She was usually very quiet in her demeanor, but if her indignation was once roused, i was no easily quelled . . . But even though I did not confide in my grandmother and even evaded her vigilant watchfulness and inquiry, her presence in the neighborhood was some protection to me. (p. 28)

Linda had another protector, her great-aunt: "At night I slept by the side of my great-aunt, where I felt safe. He was too prudent to come into her room. She was an old woman and had been in the family for many years" (p. 3).

The paradoxes of the slave system were many. Young girls were exploited, yet older female slaves were sometimes protected, mostly for their role as experienced caretakers. There was a myriad of ways mothers, grandmothers, aunts, and friends protected the female slaves when possible, negotiating to buy their freedom, infanticide, succumbing to sexual exploitation, and death or murder, if necessary, to offer some relief. The will to survive was ever-present.

In addition, in resisting the will of the slave master and other oppressive tactics of the system, the Black females would often turn to the residues of their African culture. Africans are a very spiritual people; they have always believed in a higher being than themselves. Their strong belief in spiritual strength is manifested many ways in times of stress. Linda Brent tells about her assurance after praying for her children, husband, family, home, and friends. Although being forbidden to assemble, the strength that her deep abiding faith engendered demonstrates, broadly, an African tradition.

In Kesha Yvonne Scott's *The Habit of Surviving* (1991), she calls upon Black women to develop new strategies, because the future generations are asking different questions. Too long have we been surviving in isolation. The healing rituals so prevalent in African communities are absent in American society, and we have been striving to operate without them; reinventing ourselves again and again.

The beginning of the task is to reconsider the way we think about gender-based analysis of the social, cultural, racial, sexual, and heterosexist exploitation of Black women as Blacks, women, and Americans. The beginning of the task is to acknowledge the limitations of conventional thought in these areas. The beginning of the task is to create the safety for Black women to cry, to make the movement inside, to jar the survival instincts and spiritual intuition. Then we can model for other women a truly revolutionary process and frame our own social action around our own agenda for personal and political change. (p. 22)

This is hard work and we have paid, and are still paying, the price with increased heart attacks, depression, addictions, and various other maladies. We can no longer just save ourselves or our communities; our African roots show us how to do both, and we must repossess these skills. In *Sisters of the Yam*, bell hooks (1993, p. 161) talks about the need for communities of resistance being the healing place for Black people. We see such a community created by Sula and Nel, by their friendship, in Toni Morrison's *Sula* (1973):

Except for an occasional leadership role with Sula, Nel had no aggression. Her parents had succeeded in rubbing down to a dull glow any sparkle or sputter within her. Only with

Sula did that quality have free rein, but their friendship was so close they, themselves, had difficulty distinguishing one's thoughts from the other's. They never quarreled, those two, the way some girlfriends did over boys, or competed against each other for them. In those days a compliment to one was a compliment to the other; and cruelty to one was a challenge to the other. (p. 72)

This passage points out the need for intimacy and its liberating results. Nel could live out her fantasies through Sula, who always did what she wanted to do, regardless of restrictions; she felt nurtured and safe. This safety is similar to instances where African women bonded together in ways that were empowering. There is so much that is misunderstood about African spirituality, but the connection with ancestry is always one of guidance and deeper understanding. The inhuman treatment of slaves at this time caused many to turn to the familiar for guidance, a way of repossessing cultural values. Steve Biko in his essay, "Some African Cultural Concepts" (1993, p. 87), states: "We had our community of saints. We believed—and this was consistent with our views of life—that all people who died had a special place next to God. We felt that a communication with God could only be through these people."

Linda Brent uses this resource in her times of peril:

For more than ten years I had frequented this spot, but never had it seemed to me so sacred as now. A black stump, at the head of my mother's grave, was all that remained of a tree my father had planted. His grave was marked by a small wooden board, bearing his name, the letters of which were nearly obliterated. I knelt down and kissed them, and poured forth a prayer to God for guidance and support in a perilous step I was about to take. As I passed the wreck of the old meeting house where, before Nat Turner's time, the slaves had been allowed to meet for worship, I seemed to hear my father's voice come from it, bidding me not to tarry till I reached freedom or the grave, I rushed on with renovated hopes. My trust in God had been strengthened by that prayer among the graves. (p. 93)

Black women would never have been able to survive under the perils of the slave system in America had it not been for their creativity in survival and coping skills. Through literature we can see a myriad of examples. Relying upon oral tradition, Black women have relished female griots (tribal musician-entertainers) and sister talks they have not always bothered to write down. However, the connections were ways of confirming tactics of resisting alien values and cultures. Picture the babies who were thrown off the slave ships because the mothers did not want to subject their children to the dehumanization of that kind of life. Even after being born in the system, mothers sought ways to protect their children and themselves. In Toni Morrison's *Beloved* (1987), the mother is tormented by the ghost of the child she chooses to destroy, not because she was not loved, but because she was beloved. There are a host of other examples, but the main reason these women resisted is that they understood that there had to be a better way. Handling pain can sap one's creative strength, causing confusion and reliance upon unorthodox methods. In Africa, girls are encouraged to endure the pain of the clitoridectomy because it is symbolic of withstanding all the trials and tribulations of life. John S. Mbiti states, in *African Religions and Philosophy* (1969, p. 120):

The physical pain, which the children are encouraged to endure, is the beginning of training them for difficulties and suffering that will come later in life. Endurance of physical and emotional pain is a great virtue among Akamba people, as indeed it is among other Africans, since life in Africa is surrounded by much pain from one source or another.

CONTEMPORARY COPING METHODS

Terry McMillan's novel, *Waiting to Exhale* (1992) offers insight into the plight and stress of urban America. Four women, all different in their perceptions of life, but able to cling to one another because of solid acceptance. They took care of one another whenever there was a need. After having a heart attack, Gloria heard familiar voices—Bernadine, Savannah, and Robin. Now it seemed like everybody was rubbing different parts of her body; her legs, feet, arms, and shoulders. But her feet were still cold. Why were her feet so cold?... "I think we're all responsible for her," Bernadine said. "She's our sister. Please tell us she's going to be all right." The doctor looked at all three women. He knew Bernadine was lying. But, he was used to this (p. 366).

A study by Mary Beth Snapp (1992) of 100 Black women and 100 white women in the Memphis, Tennessee, and looking at area occupational stress, showed that middle-class Black women received more social support than working-class white women. This story depicts this reality in that Black women seem to seek out the necessary stress relievers to fit their particular situation.

These questions were asked of women in the study: "Do levels of occupational stress and social support for one's career from family, friends and co-workers vary by race, class background, supervisory status, marital status and parental status?" "What are the relationships among social structure, occupational stress, social support and depression?" The findings indicate that

the black women from middle class backgrounds report much higher levels of family support, on the average, than the other groups of women. One my speculate that because many of the parents of these black women were upwardly mobile, they may be better providers of social support, appreciating the hard work required to overcome racial obstacles on the job, understanding their daughters' professional or managerial careers, and wanting to give their children the support they may have lacked for their own careers. (p. 51)

In McMillan's *Waiting to Exhale*, we see the mothers in the story being very supportive and concerned with the lives of their daughters, who are all professionals. Black motherhood has served to increase the strength of Black women; their mothers know the way and are not modest in passing this information on to heir daughters. Sometimes it is the arrangement of protection, as in the case of Janie Crawford in Zora Neale Hurston's *Their Eyes Were Watching God*, or it may be the stern instruction Maya Angelou remembers receiving in *I Know Why the Caged Bird Sings*, when her mother insisted that she nurture her child even though she was a child herself. Black mothers had to teach their daughters about life because they were their primary teachers. Angelou talks about the will to survive:

The black female is assaulted in her tender years by all those common forces of nature at the same time that she is caught in the tri-partite crossfire of masculine prejudice, white illogical hate and black lack of power. The fact that the adult American Negro female emerges a formidable character is often met with amazement, distaste and even belligerence. It is seldom accepted as an inevitable outcome of struggle won by survivors and deserves respect if not enthusiastic acceptance. (p. 231)

In critiquing this work, Joanne M. Braxton, in *Black Women Writing Auto-biography* (1989), believes that Angelou's coping mechanism was a direct result of the community of black women who nurtured her, building her self-confidence through cultural traditions (p. 197). Because of this, Braxton believes that a triple consciousness exists for the Black woman because "she knows who she is, where she comes from and what the source of her strength has been" (p. 13). This knowledge comes most commonly from gender-specific instances, like the friendships described by Terry McMillan. Bernadette, one of the protagonists of *Waiting to Exhale*, began to recount parts of her life after her husband told her that he wanted a divorce to marry a white woman. She realized that she had given up her personal power for him and their children, and when she began to resist, their relationship deteriorated. Her hairdresser suggested that she get involved in something worthwhile:

She belonged to Black Women on the Move, a support group that held workshops for women who wanted to do more with their lives than cook, clean and take care of the kids; for women who weren't moving, but wanted to move; for women who had already achieved some measure of success, but wanted to be more than role models, who were willing to make the time to do something for black folks whose lives, for whatever reason, were in bad shape. (p. 32)

Communalism is part of the African tradition. It was effective, and remains so, as explained in Paula Giddings's book, *When and Where I Enter* (1984, p. 7). She explains the difference between white and African American female groups: "Black women, many of them cramped for lack of opportunity, had frustrations too. But theirs were based on problems of the race rather than those of their particular class. The fact was, they understood that their fate was bound with that of the masses."

Being bound with the masses were also meant that the masses would not always understand one's longings. Therefore, African American women cope, sometimes, by silence and waiting. Hurston paints Janie Crawford as one who waited for self-fulfillment and love, but her spirituality helped her to persevere:

Her image of joy tumbled down and shattered. But looking at it she saw that it never was the flesh and blood figure of her dreams. Just something she had grabbed up to drape her dreams over. In a way she turned her back upon the image where it lay and looked further. She had no more blossomy openings dusting pollen over her man, neither any glistening fruit where the peals used to be. She found that she had a host of thoughts she had never expressed to him, and numerous emotions she had never let Jody know about. Things packed up and put away in parts of her heart where she could never find them. She was saving up feelings for some man she had never seen. She had an inside and an outside now, and suddenly she knew no to mix them. (p. 68)

However, in her waiting there is sporadic comforting from Phoebe, a friend who serves as the audience for the story, and by another woman who expresses empathy with her situation:

Jamie went down and the landlady made her drink some coffee with her because she said her husband was dead, and it was bad to be having your morning coffee by yourself. "Yo' husband gone tuh work dis mornin', Ms' Woods? Ah seen him go out uh good while uh go. Me and you kin be comp'ny for one 'nother, can't us?" "Oh yes, indeed, Mis' Samuels. You puts me in de mind uh mah friend back in Eatonville. Yeah, you'se nice and friendly jus' lak her." (p. 112)

Friendship has always been a very important part of the lives of females, but for black women especially so, and in this instance we see the selectivity of Janie Crawford, which illustrates that all friends are not equal. Friendships are also forged by Black women in order to write, as Hurston aligned herself with philanthropist Mrs. Rufus Osgood Mason to understand her research, and Harriet Wilson used Maria Childs to confirm her abilities as a writer in her book.

WRITING AND COPING

Writing is also another way of coping for Black women (and all women), and of providing a way of economic support for children. While, early on, the art of writing was the primary quest of males, women had to find a way to uncover their voices. During the abolitionist period, Black women had to endure racism and sexism as it pertains to writing. In the slave narratives, their voices had to be authenticated by white women and men, but they continued to speak through autobiographies, travel journals, poems, newspaper articles, and speeches. One of the main concerns of these women was the welfare of their children. Harriet Wilson, on the first page of her introduction to Our Nig (1983, p. xii), writes:

In offering to the public the following pages, the writer confesses her inability to minister to the refined and cultivated the pleasure supplied by abler pens. It is not for such these crude narrations appear. Deserted by kindred, disabled by failing health, I am forced to some experiment which shall aid me in maintaining myself and child without extinguishing this feeble life.

The sorrow song aesthetic comes forth in this appeal to the higher level of the public consciousness. While the tone is distressed, it is not hopeless. Writing was a way of coping and, at the same time, continuing to move forward for

Wilson. The sorrow song tone of writing demonstrates the way the slave narratives used Christianity to balance insult and truth. One needed the support of the white audience, while at the same time it was necessary for society to hear the clear voice of slavery. In this regard also, writing was cathartic.

Looking at women in African, it is evident that they were not always lauded for their accomplishments, even though they may have been lofty. However, they were never deterred from moving toward goals of freeing other women. In Patricia W. Romero's *Life Histories of African Women* (1991), she outlines the lives of seven women from various geographical regions, classes, and lifestyles, suffering the peculiar cultural limits of their era, yet maintaining the dignity and perseverance needed to raise children, establish schools for girls, and break cultural barriers when deemed necessary. In Beverly Mack's chapter, "Hajiya Ma'daki: A Royal Hausa Woman," we see the transitional changes in the Nigerian government and its effect on women. Ma'daki is the granddaughter of a non-Muslim Ha'be slave, daughter of a royal concubine, and became royal wife to a devout Fulani emir (known for political and religious authority). She became acquainted also with central figures in the British colony who were shapers of the lives of her people, such as Captain Frederick Lugard and Flora Shaw. Even though the ancient customs of political and cultural power relegated to women were abandoned with the Muslim Fulani influence, Hajiya Ma'daki used her cloak in resisting the status quo and established a school for girls. Education has always been the key for liberation in the eyes of Africans and African Americans.

Ma'daki's life spanned the period from strict Hausa customs to Muslim practices, and then accommodated Western technology, yet she was able to cope consistently:

Hajiya Ma'daki's life has spanned these significant historical, political and social spheres of influence since her birth, which almost coincided with the arrival of the British in Northern Nigeria. A daughter of Kano royalty, she soon became a royal wife in the nearby emirate of Katsina, thus in her life time officially representing each of two historically rival emirates. During her formative years as a young wife in Katsina, Hajiya Ma'daki witnessed her husband Dikko's concerned efforts to cooperate with the British colonists as they sought to control Northern Nigeria through indirect rule. Although colonial records are silent on the matter, Ma'daki is known to have been a trusted confidante of both Nigerian and British officials who welcomed her advice on various topics. It is clear that her husband, the Emir of Katsina, Alhaji Muhammadu Dikko, valued her perspective on events as well as her company, taking her with him during his travels. (p. 53)

One of the great confusions of the slave system for Black women had to be the cruel role they were cast into, coming from a system of respect and concern to one of inhumanity. Although Africans are transitioning in many ways to Western ideals, the positive role of African motherhood prevails.

Roots were so important that coming out of the slavery system to freedom often cast Black women in a momentary state of confusion. They were sustained by the female literary artists. Yet it is the period of the Harlem Renaissance and its strong mulatto influence that seemed to cause so much suffering and feeling of abandonment for female artists. It is not just the fact of one's color that is the primary irritant, but how one perceives that color. One might surmise that when one is disconnected from cultural roots, albeit briefly, one becomes confused and disoriented. For African and African American women, it has always been the sense of community, in its many forms, that has sustained them.

Nella Larsen's two novels, *Quicksand* (1928) and *Passing* (1929), show the futile lives of marginal women, who are products of the slave past, trapped in skin that is supposed to represent privilege, but not sufficiently pure. Helga Crane is the heroine in *Quicksand*, a middle-class professional who does not fit in, not in the southern town where she is a school teacher, not in Europe with some of her relatives, where she is looked upon as exotic, and not safely in her own skin, which is a constant reminder of her discontentedness.

She ends up marrying a Black preacher and settling for a life of emptiness. Helga Crane opted not for growth and struggle, but for defeat. She assumes this too easily. She visits her white uncle after leaving her teaching position in the South and finds a not-too-friendly reception from his wife:

"Mr. Nilssen has been very kind to you, supported you, sent you to school. But you mustn't expect anything else. And you mustn't come here anymore. It, well. frankly, it isn't convenient. I'm sure an intelligent girl like yourself can understand that." ...[However, her intelligence did not alleviate her sense of rejection.] her only impulse was to get as far away from her uncle's house and this woman, his wife, who so plainly wished to disassociate herself from the outrage of her very existence. She was torn with mad fright, an emotion against which she knew but two weapons—to kick and scream or flee. (p. 202)

Quicksand is a metaphor for no foundation and spiritual death. When Black women are estranged from their foundation and roots, they are unable to cope. Helga Crane is a woman who is rejected by her white mother and family, and never resolves this pain of abandonment. As a result, she is unable to fit in any environment. She ends up marrying a Black preacher, having babies, and resigning herself to a lifetime of unhappiness. She has no coping skills. Jessie Redmond Fauset, one of the other Black female writers of that Harlem Renaissance period, wrote four novels—*There Is Confusion* (1924), *Plum Bun* (1929), *The Chinaberry Tree* (1931), and *Comedy American Style* (1931)—plus many short stories, articles, and poems. Her theme of "passing" took on another dimension; she was more interested in using upper-middle-class blacks to prove that, with hard work and perseverance, Blacks could also make great strides. However, the heroines are narrow and frustrated. Laurentine Strange, the heroine in *The Chinaberry Tree,* is the product of an ex-slave, Aunt Saul, and her former master, Captain Halloway; they love each other passionately. At the same time that she is admired as the most beautiful as the most beautiful woman in town, she is also alienated because of her parents' strange and unusual coupling.

She can never be totally accepted. In her introduction, Fauset, who is middle class, knows how the system treats Blacks and how they feel about their heritage. She imagines the strivings of the Black male:

Finally he started out as a slave but he rarely thinks of that. To himself he is a citizen of the United States whose ancestors came over not along with the emigrants of the Mayflower, it is true, but merely a little earlier in the good year, 1619. His forbearers are to him quite simply the early settlers who played a pretty large part in making the land grow. He boasts no Association of the Sons and Daughters of the Revolution, but knows that as a matter of fact and quite inevitably his sons and daughters date their ancestry as far back as any. So quite naturally as his white compatriots he speaks of his "old Boston families," "old Philadelphians," "old Charlestonians." And he has a wholesome respect for family and education and labor and the fruits of labor. He is still sufficiently conservative to lay a slightly greater stress on the first two of these four. Briefly, he is a dark American who wears his joy and rue very much as does the white American. He may wear it with some differences, but it is the same joy and the same rue. So in spite of other intentions I seem to have pointed a moral. (p. x)

So the tragic mulatto and her estrangement from her roots represents the embryonic state of the Black woman's quest for another kind of literacy. How can she articulate this extreme experience? Earlier, Robert Stepto (1979), in his article "Narration, Authentication, and Authorial Control in Frederick Douglas' Narratives of 1845," defined the quest for literacy and freedom as the primary focus of the nineteenth-century African American novels. The early nineteenth century could represent the quest for identity, as Black women become more fully aware of their sexual, as well as racial, limitations. Because Janie Crawford, in Hurston's *Their Eyes Were Watching God*, did not become involved in the trappings of the mulatto syndrome, she was able to return to her roots, fully assured of her strength, telling her story to her friend Phoebe.

It is in later writings that we see this identity evolve more fully, with Gwendolyn Brooks winning the Pulitzer Prize for *Annie Allen* in 1950, and others developing themes away from the issues surrounding the mulatto. Maya Angelou, Nikki Giovanni, Toni Morrison, Alice Walker, and others are some of the forces who helped usher in another renaissance around the time of the Civil Rights Movement, and beyond.

The writings around the period and beyond have black women defining themselves in creative ways. Alice Walker (1983) coinage of a Black feminist as "womanist" is revealing:

Womanist—1. From womanish (opp. of "girlish," i.e., frivolous, irresponsible, not serious). A black feminist or feminist of color. From the black folk expression of mothers to female children, "you acting womanish," i.e., like a woman. Usually referring to outrageous audacious, courageous or willful behavior. Wanting to know more and in greater depth than is considered "good" for one. Interested in grown-up doings. Acting grown-up . . . Responsible. In charge. Serious . . . 3. Loves music. Loves dance. Loves the moon. Loves the spirit. Loves love and food and roundness. Loves struggle. Loves the folk. Loves herself, regardless. 4. Womanist is to feminist as purple to lavender. (xi, xii)

Womanist also serves to describe "sass" as a survival tactic of the black female. " 'Mama, I'm walking to Canada and I'm taking you and a bunch of other slaves with me.' Reply, 'It wouldn't be the first time' " (xi). Sass can be seen in a number of women's writings—for example, Toni Morrison's *Sula* and Walker's Sophie in *The Color Purple*. However, the classic example is Janie Crawford in Hurston's *Their Eyes Were Watching God,* who always maintained a sense of herself through three husbands. The turning point in the novel was the day her husband tied to humiliate her in front of others in the store and her response:

What's de matter wid you no how? You ain't no young girl to be gettin' all insulted 'bout yo' looks.
   Naw Ah ain't no young gal no mo but den Ah ain't no old woman neither. Ah reckon Ah looks mah age too. But Ah'm uh woman every inch of me, and Ah know it. Dat's uh whole lot more'n you kin say. You big bellies round here and put out a lot of brag, but 'tain't nothin' to it but yo' big voice. Humph! Talkin' 'bout me lookin' old! When you pull down yo' britches you look lak de change uh life. (p. 75)

Sass was definitely a way of coping with the pains of life for Black women. The literary criticism about and by Black female writers is revealing, as they have leaned how to cope better, and have passed it on, in the African tradition. They have coped by relishing in what they feel thy do best, not what others have said. The 600 Black women in the Myers (1991) study confirmed this in their responses and the conclusions:

When I speak of self-esteem and coping, again I mean self-esteem—coping. I am talking about a feeling of self-worth—a feeling that we are good enough. Good enough to and for whom? We are good enough to and for ourselves, our families (who count so much in our lives), and our social support systems, whose experiences are similar and whose opinions matter to us more than any others. We simply feel that we are persons of worth and respect ourselves for what we are. We do not need to be told what we should do or with whom we should identify in order to feel good enough about ourselves. (p. 61)

Catherine Fisher Collins, in her book, *Sources of Stress and Relief for African American Women*, cites the Afrocentric form of network, which involves family, work, community, and social support. The legacy of being looked upon as the other in American society forces Black women to use their ingenuity and their lives confirm the need to rely upon "other" of these resources.
   Life imitates art and Black women have plenty of art to rely upon. They cope by repossessing their roots in a myriad of ways and occasions, not because others say so, but because they know that it is the only way to return to wholeness.

REFERENCES

Angelou, M. 1969. *I Know Why the Caged Bird Sings*. New York: Random House.
Biko, Steven. 1993. Some African Cultural Concepts. In Teresa M. Redd (Ed.), *Revelations*. Needham Heights, MA: Ginn.

Braxton, J. M. 1989. *Black Women Writing Autobiography*. Philadelphia: Temple University Press.

Brent, L. 1973. *Incidents in the Life of a Slave Girl*. New York: Harcourt Brace Jovanovich.

Collins, C. F. 2003. *Sources of Stress and Relief for African American Women*. Westport, CT: Praeger Publishers.

Du Bois, W.E.B. 1969. *The Souls of Black Folk*. New York: New American Library.

Fauset, J. R. 1931. "Foreword" to *The Chinaberry Tree*, p. x. New York: Frederick A. Stokes.

Giddings, P. 1984. *When and Where I Enter*. New York: Bantam Books.

Hooks, B. 1993. *Sisters of the Yam*. Boston: South End Press.

Hurston, Z. 1990. *Their Eyes Were Watching God*. New York: Harper & Row.

Larsen, N. 1928. *Quicksand*. New York: Alfred A. Knopf.

———. 1929. *Passing*. New York: Alfred A. Knopf.

Mbiti, J. 1969. *African Religions and Philosophy*. Portsmouth, NH: Heinemann.

McMillan, T. 1992. *Waiting to Exhale*. New York: Viking Press.

Morrison, T. 1973. *Sula*. New York: Alfred A. Knopf.

———. 1987. *Beloved*. New York: Alfred A. Knopf.

Myers, L. W. 1991. *Black Women Do They Cope Better?* San Francisco: Mellen Research University Press.

Romero, P. (Ed.). 1991. *Life Histories of African Women*. London: The Ashfield Press.

Scott, K. Y. 1991. *The Habit of Surviving*. New York: Ballantine Books.

Snapp, M. 1992. "Occupational Stress, Social Support, and Depression among Black and White Professional-managerial Women." *Women and Health*, 18, no. 1.

Some, Malidoma, and Sobonfu Some. 1994. *We Have No Word for Sex*. California: Oral Traditions Archives.

Stepto, R. B. 1979. "Narration, Authentication, and Authorial Control in Frederick Douglas' Narratives of 1845." In Dexter Fisher and Robert Stepto (Eds.), *Afro American Literature*. New York: Modern Language Association of America.

Walker, A. 1983. *In Search of Our Mother's Gardens*. San Diego, CA: Harcourt Brace Jovanovich.

Wilson, H. 1983. *Our Nig*. New York: Random House.

Index

About the Editor
and Contributors

VIRGINIA A. BATCHELOR, Ph.D., is an Associate Professor in the Department of Education at Medaille College. As a professor, she inspires and instills cultural sensitivity in future educators. She cofounded Buffalo Quarters Historical Society, a community-driven organization founded in 1995 for the purpose of promoting Buffalo, New York's, significance in and contribution to American history as it relates to the Underground Railroad Movement. Dr. Batchelor's community has extended across geographical borders as she has presented her research interests internationally.

PATRICIA K. BRADLEY, Ph.D., received her bachelor's degree in nursing from Temple University. She earned both her master's degree in Psychiatric Mental Health Nursing and her doctorate in Nursing from the University of Pennsylvania. Her research interests include psychosocial issues of African American breast cancer survivors as well as other health issues of unserved groups. As an advanced practice nurse, she has demonstrated commitment and service to the unserved in her nursing research, education, and practice. Dr. Bradley is a member of Sigma Theta Tau International Honor Society of Nursing and the Oncology Nursing Society (ONS). She is nationally certified as a specialist in adult psychiatric mental health nursing and has over twenty-five years of experience as a psychiatric mental health nurse. Her work experience includes a variety of psychiatric settings such as inpatient and outpatient mental health, psychiatric consultation liaison, and private practice with adolescents and families. Currently she is an Assistant Professor of Psychiatric Mental Health Nursing at Villanova University, College of Nursing.

Dr. Bradley is also a teaching faculty member for the Cancer Prevention and Early Detection (CPED) in African Americans Institute for Nurse Educators, a program funded by the National Cancer Institute (NCI) and Oncology Nursing Society (ONS). She is a *Special Populations Investigator* (SPI) in the ACES

Program, an NCI Office of Special Populations Research (OSPR) funded program at Thomas Jefferson University Department of Behavioral Epidemiology where she recently completed a pilot study, *Preparing African American Women for Breast Biopsy*.

CATHERINE FISHER COLLINS, ED.D, earned a doctoral degree from the State University of New York's University at Buffalo, from which she also received a Master's Degree in Allied Health Education. Dr. Collins is a Nurse Practitioner graduating from the University at Buffalo's School of Nursing Nurse Practitioner program. She also holds three certifications in health education. Dr. Collins has received over thirty-five awards and citations. In 2005 she participated in and completed the Oxford Round Table at Oxford University, Oxford, England.

Dr. Collins is a respected author of several published books, including *Sources of Stress and Relief for African American Women* (2003), *The Imprisonment of African American Women: Causes, Conditions and Future Implications* (1997; winner of the 1997 Outstanding Academic and Scholarly Award), and *African American Women's Health and Social Issues* (1996). Other publications include *Parent Child Rearing Practices* (1993). She is under contract for new books that deal with women's issues.

Dr. Collins is currently an Associate Professor at State University of New York at Buffalo, Empire State College, and Adjunct at State University of New York's University at Buffalo Women's Studies Department.

RENEE BOWMAN DANIELS, M.S.S., C.S.W., is an Associate Professor in the Department of Social Work and Sociology at Daemen College. She is also an Adjunct Graduate Faculty member at the School of Social Work, State University of New York. She has published articles and chapters in professional journals among them a chapter in *African American Women's Health and Social Issues* (1996) edited by Catherine Fisher Collins. She received her undergraduate degree from Hofstra University and graduate degree from Columbia University School of Social Work.

CASSANDRA DOBSON, D.N.S.(c.), M.S.N., R.N., is administrative nurse manager, Montefiore Medical Center (MMC), Bronx, New York. In addition to teaching as an Adjunct Clinical Assistant Professor at New York University, she is a consultant on sickle cell disease for patients and their families and is the past sickle cell/comprehensive clinical care coordinator at MMC. Her expertise in practice and research is utilized on numerous committees in the hospital and at the state nurses association. She holds membership in a number of professional organizations. Ms. Dobson is completing her doctoral degree in nursing at the Columbia University School of Nursing, New York, concentrating on sickle cell pain management.

IMANI LILLIE B. FRYAR, Ph.D., is an adjunct faculty member at a historical black college, LeMoyne Owen College, in Memphis, TN, where she worked as

Associate Professor of Humanities and English Literature for seven years. Prior to that she was Assistant Professor of English and Director of a Transitional Program at the State University of New York for eleven years. The non-traditional mentoring approach to teaching in this system has informed and confirmed Dr. Fryar's approach to student learning. She is a womanist, and her special area of expertise is Black women writers. Her article, "The Aesthetic of Language: Harper, Hurston and Morrison," was published in *African-American Women Writers: An A to Z Guide*, editor Yolanda Page, Greenwood Press, 2007.

JUANITA K. HUNTER, Ph.D., is currently Professor Emeritus at the State University of New York at Buffalo and Professional Performance Review Examiner at Excelsior College. Dr. Hunter previously served as Professor in the School of Nursing from 1978 to 1998 and in 2003, as Executive Director of the Near East Side Community Health Task. Dr. Hunter was Project Director of A Nursing Center for the Homeless, a project funded by the Department of Health and Human Services, from 1987 to 1993. She has participated in several research projects related to the health needs of the homeless and authored several articles on the topic.

CHERYL HUNTER-GRANT, M.S.W., is a lifelong child advocate and sickle cell disease supporter who has worked in the field of Family Services for more than twenty-five years. Cheryl earned a master's of social work degree from Hunter College School of Social Work in New York City, and a bachelor of arts degree from Simmons College, Boston, Massachusetts.

Ms. Hunter-Grant has served as a Public Health Administrator for the New York State Department of Health coordinating Sickle Cell and Genetics Services for the Metropolitan NY Region. Following her tenure at the Health Department, Ms. Hunter-Grant directed the Programs and Health Services Divisions at the Bronx Perinatal Consortium, Inc., a state-funded Comprehensive Prenatal Perinatal Services Network. She has also worked as a Senior Program and Policy Associate with the Children's Defense Fund, New York Office, and Vice President for Marketing and Planning at Today's Child Communications, Inc. Currently she is Executive Director of the Lower Hudson Valley Perinatal Network and runs her own consulting business, IOE Total Consulting. Ms. Hunter-Grant is also a Visiting Lecturer at New York Medical College, School of Public Health, and the Cochair of the NYS Sickle Cell Advisory Consortium, Inc.

JAMESETTA A. NEWLAND, Ph.D., A.P.R.N., C.S., F.N.P., F.A.A.N.P., F.N.A.P., family nurse practitioner, is Director, Primary Health Care Associates at the Lienhard School of Nursing, Pace University, New York, where she also teaches nursing research as an Adjunct Associate Professor. A personal interest in sickle cell disease led her to study transition issues in adolescents for her doctoral dissertation. She is active in local, national, and international professional organizations and devotes time to projects for underserved populations. Dr. Newland has received numerous honors and awards and in 2005 was elected as a Fellow in the American Academy of Nurse Practitioners and the National

Academies of Practice. She is also the current Editor-in-Chief of *The Nurse Practitioner: The American Journal of Primary Healthcare.*

FREIDA HOPKINS OUTLAW, Ph.D., received her bachelor's in Nursing from Berea College, her master's in Psychiatric Nursing from Boston College, and her doctorate in Nursing from the Catholic University of America. Formerly she delivered culturally appropriate behavioral health care in a primary health setting, a University of Pennsylvania School of Nursing community practice. Presently she is the Assistant Commissioner equivalent, Special Populations, Tennessee Department of Mental Health and Developmental Disabilities. She is responsible for mental health services for children and youth, forensic, geriatric, and co-occurring (mental illness and substance abuse) individuals. Her latest publications (2005) are focused on suicide in the military and the use of the Geriatric Depression Scale with older African Americans.

LORRAINE E. PEELER, Ph.D., is Assistant Professor of Human Development at the State University of New York, Empire State College, in Buffalo, NY. She has a Ph.D. in Counselor Education from the University at Buffalo. Her research and teaching focus is counseling, social psychology, and cultural competency. She also works extensively with community-based agencies in developing programs and training that are culturally competent and sensitive to the needs of diverse groups. Dr. Peeler is a consultant to organizations in strategic planning, cultural diversity, and ethical issues in human services. She is a motivational speaker and has developed workbooks and activities to assist in raising awareness about cultural issues.

LYNNE VALENCIA PERRY-BOTTINGER, M.D., F.A.C.C., is a board-certified clinical/interventional cardiologist and President of Clinical and Interventional Cardiology PLLC. She is an honors graduate of Harvard University and Yale Medical School. She was resident and chief medical resident at Yale–New Haven Hospital and trained in cardiology at Johns Hopkins Hospital. She serves on the faculty of Columbia and Cornell Universities. She has received numerous honors and is included on many of the nation's top doctors lists. She serves on the board of various community organizations and has made national television appearances including *the Today Show* and Black Entertainment Television.

RHEA J. SIMMONS, Ph.D., is an Assistant Professor of Psychological Foundations, College of Education, State University of New York at Fredonia. She received her Ph.D. in clinical psychology from the University of Pittsburgh. In addition to being an educator, Dr. Simmons has over 20 years of experience as a clinician, advocate, and administrator in mental health services for families and children with serious emotional disturbances and mental illnesses. Dr. Simmons is the codeveloper of measures assessing coteaching practices, and a cofounder of a charter school. She has also presented at international, national, regional, and state conferences. Her research interests include informed consent, coteaching practices, integration of technology into curricula, and school-based mental health.